I0704410
HIGHEST, RAINBOW and
Michael YOGA

HIGHEST, RAINBOW and Michael YOGA

Gilead Samuel

Table of Contents

Introduction

Hello Friend! You were probably a little surprised to see instead of "Introduction" "Conclusion". This is not a mistake - with these lines I complete your past life. Before you is the final, highest technology for the development of consciousness, which will allow you to make your transition to a new era in the very near future. Technologies adapted to modern times and a secular view of them for the first time make it possible for every person to have consciousness outside the physical world. Before me is a difficult task - just to bring you to specific actions so that you understand: there is also another world, more clear and realistic than the one you are in the physical body. The task is complicated by the fact that I myself would never have believed it, if the case many years ago had not led me to such a phenomenon, which fundamentally contradicts our idea of consciousness and the space of existence.

The practice of releasing consciousness from the body, due to lightweight technical tools, reaches the widest expanses and is the most promising technology of self-development that currently exists. And the reason is simple: there is nothing more useful and interesting. This is a long-awaited evolutionary stage in the development of mankind. The explosive spread of this practice is the reason for the transition in 2012. This phenomenon can only be compared with your birth in another body, another life. It really is. But if an uncontrollable accident threw you into this world, then you can be born and live there only thanks to deliberate actions, the power of consciousness. When you at least once find yourself there, in the new world, you will understand how gray your past life was, how scarce its colors and possibilities were. And you will feel how that invisible low ceiling disappears, under which you lived all your life, only dreaming and trying to convince yourself that it does not exist. But now, however, it will not exist, and you will feel incredible lightness from understanding that the world has become a thousand times wider and you have gone beyond the boundaries of that small room in which you used to exist. Perhaps from your environment you will be one of the first to make this transition into a new era. But gradually the world will catch up with you, and it will become much easier and more interesting for everyone to live.

Buddy, I can please you: such abstract images that you just read about will not be in the book anymore. Only a small introductory information - and then specific technical actions, and nothing more. You just have to fulfill them several times in order to forever part with that slavish attitude that you don't notice yet, because everything is known in comparison. Just a few attempts - and your consciousness will gain true perception in a new, yet hidden from you world. Further more. The time has come.

Chapter first

Affordable Superpower

Buddy, I can't wait to start right away with the specific technical actions that you need to perform in order to separate consciousness from the body, so that you become a representative of a new civilization. But I am literally forced to slow down in order to first bring you up to speed a little, so that you better understand what it is all about, who I am in myself and why I have the right to talk about it. I must also give you some preliminary advice, so that your practice will be more successful due to the correct approach to business.

So the practice will begin a little later, and there will be nothing else besides it, but first try to carefully deal with the phenomenon itself, which will allow you, without exaggeration, to exist in two worlds.

Higher yoga and transition.

Yoga of Consciousness

Since the time of the Indus civilization (3300-1700 BC), about

What were the historical artifacts, the main goal of yoga was the development of consciousness. The body has always been only one of the auxiliary tools in achieving this goal. Whatever branch of the ancient Eastern civilizations you take, everywhere the foundations are based on one supreme practice, often hidden behind seven seals or requiring decades of preparation. Its essence is to bring consciousness beyond the limits of the physical body. For example, this is the eighth and highest stage of yoga - the state of samadhi (samadhi) or dream yoga. Why did ancient people and modern yogis of the highest level need it? You will be amazed, but they take this practice as training for dying. They believe that after physical death, before a new meaningless reincarnation, we find ourselves in a special state - burgundy being. But usually we cannot keep consciousness in it and that is why we find ourselves back on Earth in a new incarnation. So, if during life you train to take consciousness out of the body and at the same time maintain full awareness of what is happening, this will help to control the process after death and, finally, stop rebirth and reunite with the Universe.

Don't be afraid, my friend, it's not so scary. We live in a modern world, we have modern views and modern technologies. Honestly, I personally do not know what will happen after death and how much this practice really has to do with it, according to ancient yoga. But I know how to do it, bypassing the jungle of theories, modern and ancient prejudices. Now you don't need years of preparation. Now you don't have to be a religious orthodox. Now the separation of consciousness from the body is a matter of technology.

And the point is not only that you will soon find yourself out of your body, but also that all this is of practical importance for modern man. First, believe me, you have never experienced anything more amazing in your life and you will not survive it. Secondly, it is a way to travel to any corner of the universe and meet with any people, including the dead. Thirdly, it is an opportunity to receive information. Fourth, it is an incredible opportunity for self-healing. Fifthly, it is the destruction of all barriers for the disabled, including those who are bedridden. Now they can do anything! And everything that I just briefly listed is only the smallest fraction of what we will discuss in detail. Keep in mind, this is not some kind of imagination, idea or fantasy. It is not just that the ancient people associated this phenomenon with death. Otherwise, you will not think how bright it is in its essence. And certainly not from some imaginary image, hefty men immediately try to return from there, almost emptying their intestines from fear. Every second experiences horror at the first experiences, as it breaks all ideas about life, the self-preservation instinct works. Moreover, you probably heard about near-death experiences during near-death experiences? Departure from the body, the operating room, the tunnel ... Oh, my friend, we are just talking about this, but without subsequent death and with intentional achievement. By the way, not only the ancient yogis were fond of this practice. In its modern form, this is the same as the so-called out-of-body travel, astral projections, and even to some extent lucid dreams. But now - no nonsense and empty talk.

May history forgive me, may you forgive me, my friend, but I will use the modern terms "phase", "phase state", which unite all these phenomena into one whole, including uniting all ancient concepts. We will talk about terminologies a little later, but you must understand that I have no other choice. Since we are talking about a new era in the development of mankind, about the transition to a new level of being, we need modern concepts adapted for wide social strata, beyond the stereotypes and prejudices that have overgrown all the previous ones. Well, and most importantly, whether you are an inveterate materialist, whether you are an orthodox esotericist - it does not matter. I don't care how you explain it to yourself and how it relates to your world. You can think of it as the exit of the soul from the body. You may think that these are super-realistic hallucinations. It doesn't matter. It is important to me that you succeed as soon as possible. And the technologies that you will receive in this book are so perfected by thousands of my students that you will still survive the exit of consciousness from the physical body, no matter what you think about it. Practice is what will finally connect us all. She is clear. You just try.

Evolution 2012. The era of a new civilization

The purpose of this book is not just to give individuals a new practice. The purpose of this book is to open your eyes to the fact that the world is many times wider than it may seem. Buddy, this is about you. You are capable of more, and when you understand and experience this, your world will change. You will become different. Your attitude to the world around you will change dramatically. Do not be afraid of this word, you will be born again. You will become happier and richer in every way. But let's imagine that there will be many like you. And more. And further. The practice of phase states in global expansion will make a kind of revolution in human consciousness. It's not just about those crazy applications. It's not just about how amazing the experience is in itself. To a greater extent, I mean precisely the evolution of human thinking and consciousness. Is it a joke when each of us will understand that there is a world in ordinary physical reality, where there are rules and restrictions, and there is another world, with completely different rules, without restrictions and with incredible possibilities? And it is available every day, and you can apply and get from it everything that is missing here and now! When we know this, not me and you, but everything around, life will become much calmer, more pleasant and interesting. Not a bad dream, is it? Start with yourself and the world will be the same, buddy. This is evolution. The transition of consciousness to a different level of perception and even being! We are accustomed to only talk about it and dream about it, but it is here, in front of you, just take it and learn. Moreover, this evolution itself, and specifically in relation to the propagation of phase states, is a completely inevitable phenomenon. With our culture and form of being, we seem to have occupied one basin in an endless valley, created a dam and lived in peace. But a trickle of endless development began to fill the entire space of our isolated basin. And the moment came when the water simply rushed over the side of the dam into that vast space behind it. This space is a phase that has only one limitation - your desire. And we can't help falling into it. We simply have nowhere else to develop ...

Surprisingly, the independent practice discussed in this book is only the first link in a more global development. Technology will follow consciousness. They will master this phenomenon, and Mindnet, that same Matrix, will be born. The foundation is already there - the space of the phase, and the very existence of the phenomenon. In fact, you can already dive there on your own, thus touching the incredible future.

You ask, where was this phase before? Why did people take little interest in this, albeit under other names? The answer is simple. Previously, this was incomprehensible to the average person and there were no available technologies. The dominance of occult terms was a barrier to the emergence of the phenomenon in the broad masses. The approach that you will find in this book is so universal that it unites the same occultists even with absolute materialists. Now it does not matter at all what views of the world you profess. There is a practice that you can't argue with. And this practice is like a miracle that we all stopped dreaming about when we grew up. And it is. Here it is. All survivors of the phase state in a profound form unequivocally affirm that this is the most powerful experience in their life. Nothing compares to this. We won't go far. Let's take me. Do you know why I devoted my whole life to this cause, as soon as I accidentally ran into it when I was still a teenager? Yes, I just realized that this is the most incredible thing that can be. I just have never seen or experienced anything more interesting and unusual in my life. Nothing else gives so many emotions and application opportunities. Believe me, I don't need to mock myself. I only do what gives me pleasure. And in all my life I have never met anything stronger and better. A little later you will understand what I mean ...

In 2012, all of humanity expects another end of the world. We just have a habit. feature of human thinking. There hasn't been a year in the past hundred years that someone, somewhere, hasn't been expecting this event. But now there are more reasons for its onset than ever before. Observing the speed with which the secular approach to the practice of separation of consciousness from the body (that is, the practice of the phase) is spreading, I can say for sure that this is precisely what will cause the end of the old era and the beginning of a new era of human existence. There are several reasons for this, with which it is difficult to argue even for a stubborn materialist (however, this is exactly what I myself am).

Firstly, that secular, technical and pragmatic approach to a long-known phenomenon makes it completely accessible in the understanding and practice of every person. Naturally, esotericists have always been interested in him. But now they are more interested in people who do not really believe in God, even in the concept of the soul. But before, with other approaches, they considered all this nonsense, and the people who do this - psychos. Moreover, everyone finds a lot of useful things in the phenomenon, and as a result, all this makes the propagation of the phase on a planetary scale only a matter of the near future. The turning point comes in 2012. Secondly, in addition to global distribution, this phenomenon also carries a fundamentally new form of being. We are used to living in only one flat world. And now it turns out that this is only a small part of our possibilities, the most limited of them. And this is not empty talk (which I myself can not stand). This is a real and, most importantly, accessible practice for everyone, which has already been proven by countless people. Now everyone will perceive the world in a completely different way. Everyone will live in two worlds, which we could only dream of before.

And when this happens to everyone, it will be a revolutionary new era of being, reflected in all aspects of the physical and parallel worlds. Dear friend, we can discuss for a long time why the topic of transition to a new level of being in 2012 is directly related to the practice of the phase. But this is redundant. A little more time will pass, and you will not only understand this, but you yourself will take a step into a new era. Maybe this is a little unexpected, because everyone thinks that this leap will happen on its own, but it turns out that you need to make an effort. But that's the reality. Of course, you yourself will choose: to stay in the old world or become a representative of a new civilization. However, to be honest, I can't even imagine how you can resist such a temptation. We've all matured for this. There is only one step left.

The term "phase", "phase state"

Buddy, so that you do not get confused in the future and do not get angry at me for a new word, I explain several reasons that prompted me to introduce it.

The generic term Phase is not yet another name for a well-known phenomenon, as many mistakenly believe. The fact is that this phenomenon itself has too many names that mean different things. These are astral travel, out-of-body experiences, lucid dreams and a number of lesser known ones. In my opinion, these phenomena have much in common, and their division into different components in the 21st century has become widely contested, as the prevalence of the practice has reached the global level. Previously, when there were some theories, these phenomena were attributed to different things. But now any person in practice will easily confirm that the properties of space are the same for all these experiences.

Since the previous statement may seem controversial to someone (probably who has not conducted relevant personal experiments), we will not dwell on this in detail. One way or another, any state in which you are fully aware of yourself, but at the same time you understand that you are outside the sensations of your physical body, is a phase. At the same time, you do not feel the real body, but the felt body is in the same real world in terms of perception, as in wakefulness. As can be seen, this condition fits all previously known terms.

Stereotypes

Of course, my friend, I could choose one of the existing terms, attach my views to it and promote it in this way. But what will come of it when all the known terms have been occupied for a long time by esoteric circles, which have created for them a far from so positive and understandable image? Tell an ordinary person "astral" - he will say that you need to be treated. Say "out-of-body experience" - he will say that you have read something incomprehensible. Say "lucid dream" - he will say, well, a dream, well, a lucid one, and what is it about, and why is it needed? But this has nothing to do with sleep, either in essence or in quality. Say "phase" - he will ask what is it? And here you are clear to him and from a pragmatic position, explain the essence of the phenomenon, since a person does not have stereotypes regarding this term. This term is not corrupted by strange people with strange outlooks on life. And if we are talking about the mass dissemination of the practice of the phase, then only such an approach is needed. As experience shows, if a phenomenon is presented, for example, as an astral plane, then no more than 10% of people will be interested in it. The situation is similar with other terms. But if you present the phenomenon as a phase, then up to 80% of people begin to be interested in it. So it is this approach that will allow humanity to move to a different level of development, making this practice an everyday occurrence. With the old terms, this is simply not possible.

Ambiguity of concepts

Not only are the old terms defeated by stereotypes among the broad masses, but the same terms are understood differently. If we are talking about your hyper-realistic feelings when traveling in an incredibly bright world, then the same concept of "exit to the astral plane" is not always given the same interpretation! Most of the time, they mean simple imaginary journeys in a relaxed state, something like visualization or representation. One term, but these things do not even touch! One needs to learn and know how to do it, and the other - sat down and flew ...

The nature of experiences

I have already spoken about the full reality of experiences more than once, and I will emphasize this more than once, because this is the most important characteristic of experiences in a phase. It is worth paying special attention to this, since most people are sure of the fuzziness of sensations and often assume that this is something like an ordinary dream. Such conclusions are undoubtedly wrong and misleading, which in turn affects the whole attitude of a person to this issue. In this section of the book, I will describe all the smallest details of self-perceptions in the phase. All the misunderstandings that arise in people who are suddenly confronted with the separation of mind and body are mainly related to the full reality of everything, down to the smallest detail. When you suddenly

suddenly take off into the air and hover under the ceiling, if this is the first time with you, then keep confidence in the flight of a real body, and not some phantom experience. And when you are convinced of the invariable position of the physical body, then there will be no doubts about the real separation of the soul, and you can even think about death coming at the moment and get very scared.

So, the most fundamental thing is the complete lack of connection with the real body and all its sensations. While in the phase, you can only guess about the existence of a physical body lying somewhere on the bed. You do not feel on which side it lies, how the arms and legs are located, whether there is light or dark, and even more so, you do not feel the orientation of the body in space. However, do not worry about the possibility of someone harming your body during such a state. This is impossible. It is also a mistake to believe that the reality of experiences lies only in the reality of the visible image - vision, although this is the most important thing. In everyday life, we receive 80-90% of all the information around us through the organs of vision, even during a conversation, we use our eyes to decipher the true meaning of words, perceiving non-verbal gestures, which contain at least 40% of information. Often we do this without suspecting, on a subconscious level, so many may be surprised by the numbers. In the phase, vision plays an equally important role. This is the most important and strong side of experiences. The visible image is so real that it is impossible to get used to it, and at first it leads to extraordinary delight and even to frenzy and shock. I have thousands of experiences, but until now I often only look at the surroundings in the phase, not believing myself that I really see it.

It is worth noting in advance that all sensations are not only the same as in the physical world, but, to some extent, even more real in perception. At least, this is how it turns out, if we judge all this from a scientific point of view, because it turns out that all sensations arise directly in the cerebral cortex without a relatively long journey along the nerves from receptors, which slightly distort reality. It can be said that feelings in the phase are even more vivid than in real life. They are livelier, clearer, which gives extraordinary pleasure and makes it possible to experience some events very vividly, including pleasure and even true pain. This applies to all feelings.

By virtue of the foregoing, even simple sight allows you to get pleasure there, and it is generally impossible to overestimate the importance of this for the blind. It is not only the clarity of the image that is striking, but also its detail, detail. This is not a computer game where, when approached, objects become angular, as if they were made of cubes. There you can take any object, bring it to your eyes and examine everything, even what cannot be seen in the real world. It's fantastic, but you can go to the bookcase, get any book and read it; you can see the skin cells on your own or someone else's hands, etc. It is worth noting the amazing range of colors, which in life you can only dream of. There is no limit to vision - this is confirmed every time. And you, my friend, will face this more than once.

The sensation of movement is very important for those who want to practice the phase, as it is one of the most spectacular aspects of the possible activity. Indeed, where else can you experience a fall from a height of a hundred meters without a parachute? You can really get scared and not decide to jump, because the feelings will be the same. Every time you walk there, fly or fall, everything is the same as it could be in the physical world. As is commonly believed, a person almost more than anything in the world dreams of learning to fly; we are all not indifferent to this dream and always rejoice if we manage to fly in a dream. But in the phase it is many times more real... Therefore, one should not be surprised that simple movement in the air gives pleasure, especially since it is not limited by anything. You can fly at the speed of light, change direction abruptly, experience overloads - all that is almost impossible in life.

When mentioning real sensations in the phase, one should not forget about taste sensations. For people who don't have tasty foods for financial or dietary reasons, this section is of great importance. I can judge this from my own experience: I had to experience hunger for both of the above reasons. Since childhood, I know very well what tasty and tasteless food is and what its complete absence is. Therefore, the ability to quench my thirst for food in the phase still plays a big role for me. Of course, I'm more thirsty psychological. How nice it is to at least occasionally experience the pleasure of a delicious product during a diet, and with experience you can learn how to create menus that come to mind.

In the phase, all sensations are possible and real in terms of experiences, and there are even those that cannot be experienced in real life. The sensation of pain is no exception, but it is an undesirable manifestation for most. It arises only through their negligence or inexperience, because all feelings are controlled. Of particular note is the reality of tactile sensations and sensations of pleasure. For some, this will be the most important aspect of experiencing the phase. So, if you decide to touch a tree during the phase, you will feel all the smallest roughness of its bark, temperature, density. Just as vividly, you will feel the touch on the human body... And even more - you can indulge in love pleasures with all the accompanying sensations, which are also brought to their logical end. And it can be even brighter than in reality, and more than once. And if you take into account that you choose partners, and the choice is limited only by your desire ...

In general, I just want to show that there all the sensations are the same and even more vivid than in everyday life. And while we are talking about what you are used to feeling here, and there are still a lot of other things. For example, have you ever wondered how a dragonfly feels and controls its wings?

The nature of the phenomenon

Perhaps, dear friend, now I will disappoint you. I am not going to go into details about the nature of this phenomenon. Do you know why? I don't really know her. I am competent in how to master the phase, how to manage it and apply it, but I have only my personal views on the very nature of this phenomenon. I could voice them, if not for one thing: at least once I have already changed my views to diametrically opposed ones ... Am I mistaken now? I understand that when there is little practice, there is nothing left but to talk about theories. Therefore, you can meet a lot of authors who have a primitive practical level, but 90% of the books are devoted to stories about what it is. I will not do it. The book is "not rubber", otherwise there is not enough space to talk about theories.

There are a few basic views, and while reading you will understand which camp I belong to, but it does not matter. No matter what anyone thinks, there is a unifying moment: practice. The uniqueness of the phase lies precisely in this - it unites both inveterate mystics and materialists who do not even believe in the human soul. Isn't that what we could only dream of? So which of the most common views dominate? The most ancient theory, often associated with the concept of "astral", is the journey of the soul in some kind of parallel world, the world of spirits. A more modern view, more related to the term "out-of-body travel", is the exit of the soul from the body into the everyday world. By the way, you just can't avoid thinking about it when you're experiencing a phase for the first time. This is the most accurate description of the feeling of experience, which is why I often use this term myself.

Well, the most dynamically developing theory says that this is all a hyper-realistic state of the brain, a kind of dissociative experience. That is, despite the monstrous reality and the complexity of building the world in which you find yourself, all this is only in your head and does not go beyond it. It should also be said that most people combine all these views. In practice, it looks like they relate different experiences of the phase to different phenomena, based on some indicators. But believe me, my friend, the properties of space are always the same.

Whatever this state may be by its nature, it exists, is accessible to everyone, has an applied value and is represented by me as a "phase".

One way or another, friend, in no case do not make the mistake that I and thousands of others have gone through, do not draw conclusions from your own thoughts, words or other people's books. Draw conclusions about the nature of the phenomenon only on the basis of your personal practical experience. This is the only authority that should be trusted. Don't even believe a single word I say. Everything is just a note. Reality is what you will confirm in practice, repeat again and experimentally verify. And only so.

If you have no practice, but have heard or read a lot about this phenomenon, then I can tell you this not very pleasant thing: almost everything that you think about it has nothing to do with reality. You know, on my way there are often people who try to prove that I am wrong about something. Foaming at the mouth, they are proving something to me, a person who has dedicated his life to this since childhood, has many thousands of experiences of the phenomenon, conducted thousands of experiments in it, knows personally a whole army of practitioners, taught this to a myriad of people. But when I ask them where they got all this from and how wide their own experience is, it almost always turns out that everything is taken from some books, and the experience itself has not yet been ... Isn't it funny?

Availability and types of techniques

And here I will please and reassure you; this phenomenon is available to absolutely everyone. Yes, it is easier for someone to master the phase, for someone it is more difficult, but it is definitely achievable for any person. You just need to do the right techniques at the right time. It is not in vain that I combined accessibility with the types of techniques for entering the phase. The fact is that it was the wrong techniques and those performed at the wrong time that made this phenomenon a rarity, which is even hard to believe. Roughly speaking, for many years people tried to get into the next room, breaking through the concrete wall with their foreheads. Someone had a straw wall, someone had an iron head, but most were wasting their time and effort. But it was possible to open the door and calmly go through ... It is the knowledge of the presence of this very door that breaks the age-old fetters and makes this practice widespread. However, I want to say right away: everything that will be discussed in this book is the so-called autonomous techniques, that is, we will not talk about any external influences. Devices, special pills, work in pairs, and even more so all sorts of cacti, mushrooms and pills, we omit. I believe that development occurs only when you do everything yourself. Moreover, no matter how hard the manufacturers of all sorts of devices and sounds, I have not yet seen a single stable practitioner who would use them. And if some chemicals allow you to experience similar sensations, then, as a rule, there is no control, and this is simply harmful.

What are we going to talk about, my friend? We will analyze three main types of techniques for entering the phase state: indirect techniques, awareness in a dream, direct techniques. Indirect techniques are actions against the background of awakening, immediately after it. And it doesn't matter how much you slept: an hour, all night or five minutes. The main thing is that you woke up and immediately started quoting indirect techniques. These are the most simple and working techniques. This is the same door to another room.

Awareness in a dream is generally attributed by many to a different practice, but in reality it is the same entrance to the phase, but not from consciousness, but from the process of dreaming. In action, this happens in such a way that during sleep you suddenly clearly understand that everything around is a dream and your consciousness becomes the same as now: full and clear. Techniques are not the most manageable, but affordable.

Direct techniques - this is exactly what is why the phenomenon itself was considered inaccessible for a long time. Everyone stubbornly struggled to get out of the body with these direct techniques. Their essence is that you need to enter the phase from full wakefulness, not interrupted by falling asleep. That is, he lay down and immediately began to do something to get into the phase. It is useless for a beginner to start with such techniques. This is a way to spend a lot of time and effort without getting anything. And if you get it, it is very rare, once every few months. These techniques should be approached only after mastering the indirect techniques.

Example from practice:

February, 2001
I woke up at night and remembered the phase. This thought caused me a strong excitement, bordering on fear. Thanks to this, I got into a stable phase. I began to experiment with vibrations, but it was scary to disengage. Gradually, the vibrations became so strong

that I was voluntarily pushed out of my body. With difficulty overcoming fear, soared in the room. Gradually, as vision appeared, he noted how night turns into day. At one point, he stood on the floor and was frightened by the reality of what was happening. However, there was a table by the window of the room that shouldn't have been there. But I did not think about it, because I was still very excited about what was happening. Concentrating on the situation, I noticed a glass with some liquid standing on the table. The idea arose to try how real the taste sensations are. Infinitely surprised at reality, he went to the table, picked up a glass and raised it to his eyes in order to better examine it. Then he raised it uncertainly to his lips and took a sip. Oh my God!!! I didn't even expect it to be so real. There was tomato juice in the glass. I clearly felt it with my lips, tongue, sky. I truly enjoyed its taste as it passed down my throat. I felt the cold of the glass with my hands and lips - everything was indistinguishable from reality. Enjoying the taste and triumphing over what was happening, I slowly swallowed the juice and thought about the new frontiers opening before me. But I completely forgot about concentration, and there was a foul. After such an opening, the whole day the mood was great.

Ordinary story

Buddy, if you're only interested in practice, you can safely skip this section of the book. In it, I would like to talk a little about how it all started with me. If all this had not happened to me, in my life I would never have believed those people who tell how they fly out of the body. Understanding this point makes me very loyal to the skeptics regarding this issue. It's hard to say that since childhood I was somehow especially interested in magic or mysticism, but one of my favorite topics has always been UFOs and extrasensory perception. All this would be trite if everything hadn't changed dramatically on one autumn night. I was 15 years old. I just went to bed and just woke up in the middle of the night, but those were the last moments of that old life. Starting from these seconds, everything will change dramatically, and something will appear in my life that will become the core of all further existence. I did not immediately notice the strangeness of the situation. It seemed like a normal awakening, although I felt unusually alert for such a late hour and such an abrupt awakening. I tried to either roll over or scratch myself, but it didn't work. I could not move, because I was like a stone, a log. The understanding of this fact caused a sharp wave of physically palpable fear that seized and swallowed my whole being with all my thoughts and desires. Buddy, I later learned that this phenomenon is not so rare and is called sleep paralysis, stupor, sleepy catalepsy. According to my statistical observations, one out of three or four people faced this at least once in their life. Interview your friends on this topic and you can easily confirm this fact, or maybe you yourself experienced it. This phenomenon is relatively well studied by science and is not something fantastic, although you cannot say so from experience. The fact is that against the background of the so-called phase of REM sleep, when we dream, the brain blocks the signals to the physical body so that we do not convulse when we dream about how we run away from angry dogs. But sometimes it happens that the human consciousness wakes up before this blockage is turned off - and this is where something just doesn't happen with poor people.

But back to that night and to my personal story. Frightened to death, at first I still tried to move, but soon realized that I simply had no chance of doing so. I couldn't even move my little finger. Only my eyes opened and closed. The fear of the unknown experience only grew, and I finally figured out what was happening. Of course, it seems ridiculous now, but I was absolutely sure that aliens would abduct me. It was impossible to think otherwise, since I was very passionate about this topic, I dreamed about such an abduction all the time and read it many times: it almost starts like this every time. As soon as I thought about it, my thoughts were instantly confirmed - my body began to smoothly rise above the bed. My fear was indescribable! Mentally, I asked for a reprieve from the invisible beings, and I was laid back. Before I had time to take a breath, an unknown force lifted me up again, in the same petrified form. This time the movement was much more confident and purposeful. First I ended up in the center of my room, and then I was dragged to the window. To my surprise, I did not break it, but went through it. It was really amazing because I was sure that I took off physically. Pay attention, my friend, to this moment, to see how realistic these experiences are. Having flown out into the street and found myself in front of my window, seeing clear stars in the sky, I had already resigned myself to the inevitable, so I tried to calm down, but at that very moment everything immediately stopped - I suddenly found myself in bed. Later you will understand the connection between relaxation and the duration of being in the phase.

Many people after this story told me that it was a dream. But have I never dreamed? Neither before nor after have I experienced such a dream. It could just as well be called a dream if you lie down on the bed now and think that you just lay down on it in a dream. It was real.

It was the beginning. Of course, for another two years I was sure that I was abducted by UFOs, but they simply erased my memory of what happened after I was outside the window. I wasn't lying if I told you about it. It really was. At first glance, if you believe your eyes. And we believe the eyes most of all, my friend? When you get into a phase state spontaneously and do not know how to control it, something that you subconsciously expect or fear most of all begins to happen to you. That is why, when a person does not notice that he has fallen into a phase, he simply walks around the apartment, doing his usual business. He thinks he just got up. But another thing is when he immediately realizes that something very strange is happening to him.

For example, what will happen to a person if he read many times that UFOs are abducted at night under similar circumstances, moreover, he dreamed about it? It will begin to happen, and just as real in sensations, as if it were happening for real, and sometimes even more realistic. So my hobby played such a strange joke with me that changed my whole life. What would happen if I thought I was dying? Or if I were a deep believer?

That's right, there would be light at the end of the tunnel or God appeared to me. And this happens to people all the time. Another question is how they then interpret it ... Once having experienced it, believing your eyes, it is almost impossible to refuse the fact that everything was exactly the way it was. Unfortunately, the phase is not the place where one should treat what is happening like that, no matter how real it may be.

Friend, I want to please you again: if you have read all the previous pages and even if you throw this book away, then somewhere with a 30% probability, you will still experience an out-of-body experience within a month, maximum two ... Not necessarily follow the recommendations of such books. They themselves program for experience.

My research and books

Don't worry, my friend: stress and shock when experiencing a phase state are not essential components of it. Therefore, your first hit in the deep phase will not necessarily bring as much trouble as it did with me.

After that first incident, which unambiguously showed me that life is not such a gray thing as it already began to seem to me, there was a certain break until everything happened again. If after the first time I could no longer fall asleep for a long time, and indeed I was afraid for a long time, then everything happened in a much milder form. The reason for this was the absence of imaginary aliens. I just woke up in the same stupor. I already knew that I could just stand up or fly up in some kind of phantom body, but I was still afraid to do it.

Gradually, I began to try to get up and go in this process a little further than last time. This tactic adapted me to fear, which no longer dominated. At the same time, I was occupied with the fact that I do it myself, albeit uncontrollably. That is, if for the first time I was allegedly pulled out of the body by little green men, now there was not even a hint of them. It turned out that this is some kind of skill that can be developed. Of course, being interested in extrasensory perception, it was impossible to ignore the idea that this ability is directly related to this. Moreover, this is the most interesting of this area. And most importantly - it was a reality, and not stubborn attempts to believe in something barely perceptible and ambiguous. Not surprisingly, I began to dig through all possible literature, trying to find useful information. After all, you can find everything in books, and only the truth is written there, isn't it, my friend?

Suffice it to say that I quickly had to give up all the literature that came to hand. The reason is that every week I got better at learning a new interesting experience in practice and could easily check the statements and facts from the books. It turned out that there is very little real in them and much more long-term tricks. There was simply no point in starting from these "works". You have to go your own way. Understanding that only I myself can find answers to all questions, served as the impetus for development, which is lacking for many, especially those who are trying to turn some authors into unconditional authorities. With that in mind, I always advise people to approach things the same way. Alone with myself and my own strength, I began to literally storm this amazing state. For about 15 to 20 years, I lived only this and nothing else. I was already alone, and no one could stop me. Of course, I became somewhat asocial, but literally every day I conducted such a huge number of experiments and experiments that their result was worth any sacrifice on my part. Not only that, it was just the most interesting thing in the world. This practical onslaught brought many useful results. First, I gradually grasped how to get into this strange state intentionally, and not spontaneously. Secondly, I came to the understanding that no aliens abducted me, therefore, my friend, do not worry about my health. Thirdly, I began to understand the properties of the space where I got.

It is important that at that time the theoretical foundation was laid: understanding the technique of maintaining this state, the need to deepen it, interact with space, move and find objects in it, and much more. In addition, I was able to classify all the technical nuances, which was so lacking for a structured practice. Especially it is necessary to note the applied side. It was this moment that first of all influenced the fact that I threw away other books. For example, they described that in this state you can fly to some person and pinch him, and then in reality he will have a bruise. God only knows how many desperate attempts I made to verify this. Yes, you can find a friend there and pinch him, but then he will not remember this in reality, and there are not even hints of any bruises. You know, friend, I am the author of more than a dozen books that are not thin at all, and I can tell you that only my conscience and nothing else is responsible for the truthfulness of the content ... Even if a person has a conscience, he will be clear, he can easily make mistakes, and you can accept it as the truth in the first instance. That's why I tell you all the time: don't pay attention to theories. Only real practice is knowledge of the world. As time went on , I developed several major advantages in my techniques. One of them is that in practice I have "carved out" a large list of applied uses of this phenomenon, which can be applied by every person, having got into the phase the first time, regardless of their worldview.

Looking back at those times, I am not surprised that at the age of 20 I wrote my first book on the subject. Although it was somewhat unsightly, people liked it, and no one guessed how old its author was. But most importantly, the techniques described in it really helped people find their new body outside the shackles of the physical world. Then there were more books on various applied areas. My best book was the tenth - "Practical Textbook", which is devoid of living text and looks more like a textbook on physics than a book on the practice of self-development. The only drawback is that it is impossible to read it without being aware of the matter, why it and the book that you are now holding in your hands were born. This is a symbiosis of an interesting explanatory text and material from the same textbook.

School and its lessons

Even before writing the first book, that is, before the age of 20, I tried to teach the phase to people. But I didn't think I would ever take it seriously. When my first book came out, I immediately had a lot of fans and followers, and some of them just pestered me with requests for training. I was literally persecuted for this purpose. Often people were many times older than me and did not even suspect that they dreamed of studying with a youngster, why I did not dare to do this for a long time. Moreover, people are full of stereotypes and prejudices, which is why my external achievements in sports did not benefit me for a long time. The intelligence of athletes does not inspire respect and confidence. Frankly, in the world of sports, I have repeatedly convinced myself that there is a reason for this. But after all, the desire to be in excellent physical shape can also be considered as a level of comprehensive development of a person. So here and there, your body should be ready for anything, as well as looking great. To put it simply, for a few more years I had my own ideas about life, and the practice of the phase was its decoration. But one day everything changed dramatically. Once I looked into my mail and noticed that the question about whether I am conducting training comes almost every day from people from different parts of the planet. And so, at the age of 24, I decided to try to conduct the first classes, taking responsibility for the result. It must be said that I was the first to speak about the result, and not about interesting arguments, about such a magical phenomenon.

At first, these were two-month courses, where 90% of the students at least once in two months fell into the phase, and someone even managed to master it well during this time. Considering that some people do not believe in it at all, and some are used to the idea that it takes years to learn something, this result seemed significant to me, and it inspired me. This confirmed that the technologies developed in my youth work not only for me! It's one thing to know that people learn from books, but it's quite another thing to see it with your own eyes. In addition, I was very pleased to observe the emotions of people who received what they could only dream of: the opportunity to get into another world, whatever it was in its essence.

The effectiveness of the classes gradually grew, and after about six months , my courses became very popular. Seminars in the capital were monthly, but enrollment for them ended in two or three weeks, as there were a lot of people who had heard that you can get real practice here, and quickly enough. The most interesting thing started about two years later. You need to understand that I immediately began to consider training people as a wonderful research resource. I received an insane amount of information. In the workshops, I constantly experimented with techniques in search of the best options. As a result, the classes took the form of three-day seminars, in which up to 80% of the participants fell into the phase! Dude, this is also not a typo and not a publicity stunt. There are many witnesses to this. These results shocked me. I didn't even dream about it and never thought that it was even possible. It's funny, but if only half of the group got into the phase in two days, I was already upset. It became normal when half of the participants the very next day, after the first session, told how from one to several times they flew out, rolled out of the body or became aware of themselves in a dream. At the same time, most people initially believe that the idea itself is generally nonsense and nothing like this happens! It's simple: if it doesn't work, you're doing something wrong. This is the basic rule that allows you to achieve such results.

Don't worry my friend, you don't have to go to my School to get access to the best technology. They are all in this book. Just carefully follow what will be written in the technical sections.

Example from practice:

December, 2008
I woke up after a daytime sleep in a drowsy state and immediately tried to roll out and take off, but nothing happened. However, I felt that the state was very close

to the phase. I tried force sleep and felt my consciousness fail, and images appear before my eyes. After a few seconds, I decided to try to separate again, while thinking that, if it didn't work out, I could switch to observing images, since they are already there. However, it didn't come to that, and I was able to just stand up very easily. Vision appeared on its own immediately. He quickly brought the state to high realism by feeling the surrounding objects and looking at them. I also managed to quickly feel my whole body while creating and intensifying vibrations for guaranteed fixation in the deep phase.

There was a clearly defined plan of action related to the study of the phase, but I had been struggling with its details for several days, and right now I wanted, first of all, to use the phase just for myself, to do what I wanted most. About a week ago, in class, I told my students about the opportunity to walk next to dinosaurs, and I myself got excited about this idea, since I hadn't done anything like that for a long time. Therefore, he abandoned the previous plan of action and, closing his eyes, concentrated his attention on the tyrannosaurus rex. There was also a sense of movement. As usually happens in such cases, the transfer was longer than usual, since it was purely psychologically difficult for me to fully believe that such a thing would succeed, although it had already succeeded many times. Things like encounters with dinosaurs are not so easy to fit in the head.

Still managed to curb and concentrate, and I fell on something soft. It was land in the forest. Immediately he began to peer into the soil before his eyes and feel it. Vision almost instantly manifested and became very clear. I stood on all fours and for a while just looked at everything that was at hand. Basically, these were small sticks of various shapes, half-rotten or rotten leaves. There were also insects crawling around. Then I turned my attention to my own feelings and perceptions. I was wearing the same shorts and T-shirt as in reality. The body itself seemed unusually white. But what surprised me the most was how difficult it was to breathe. Not only was the air very saturated with extremely disgusting odors that are simply impossible to describe, but it turned out to be very hot and humid. I tried to breathe only through my nose - I felt dizzy. I tried it with my mouth - it hurt and my throat was hot. Still, I decided to breathe through my throat, as the pain was easily removed.

Pay attention to the environment. There was a forest around. The sun is almost invisible. The trees are very tall, with long straight trunks. There are many fern-like plants around, only larger than usual, almost as tall as me. In the place where I ended up - a small clearing without trees. Everything was filled with some unnatural sounds for an ordinary forest. Instead of birds singing, I heard some whistles and wheezing. Somewhere in the distance, a roar could be heard from time to time. Something constantly crunched and fell. And because of the huge bushes about thirty meters away from me, I heard a steady rustle and sometimes thumps. I immediately realized that my object was there. When I already began to itch from the constant attack, from the air and from the ground, insects of various colors and sizes unknown to me, I decided to go to the goal. While walking, he also actively peered first at his hands, then at the leaves that he plucked with his hands. Specially ran up to tree trunks. I followed the hyper-realism very carefully, as now it has become the most important factor. The vibrations also did not subside, as I constantly, from the very beginning, controlled them.

He walked over to the bushes and carefully peered behind them. There was a stream surrounded by swampy soil, from which a huge horsetail was sticking out. And in the middle of the stream stood my object, at the sight of which I almost screamed with delight. I did not do this only because I did not really want to attract his attention to myself. It could ruin everything. And the matter is not only in some fear, but also in the desire to simply look at all this miracle from the outside, to admire the beauty. I had seen a Tyrannosaurus rex at least five times before, but this one was much larger than the previous ones. Even the color was different - a little darker and with fewer spots. For some reason it looked like a female. At some point, the giant froze, apparently reacting to me. I immediately got distracted by looking at the leaves and insects on them so as not to interfere in the situation and at the same time remain in the deep phase.

I was very afraid that the phase might not be enough for more sensations, so I could not stand it and quickly ran behind the back of the tyrannosaurus. He instantly turned in my direction, but I forced myself to concentrate on the thought as best I could so that he would perceive me as a friendly object. At the risk of a phase, I even froze to program the situation. The huge head looked at me for a few more seconds and again leaned down indifferently. Looks like there was a victim. Ran up to a massive tail. Quickly seeing him close, moved to the muzzle. At the same time, being terribly afraid for the phase and its depth, he did everything to increase the vibrations. My hands touched the lizard all the time as I moved along it, dipping my ankles in the cool water. Everything was very unusual, and I did not want to be stupidly thrown into reality. The fear of the monster completely disappeared, but I began to worry a little because the phase was too deep. The incredible thought of staying here forever again treacherously overtook me. But so far I have successfully mastered the instinct of self-preservation. Touching the massive and muscular body of the lizard, I got to its front. I hadn't often seen tyrannosaurs so close and had contact with them, so it became a little funny to me from the helpless appearance of the front legs, similar to claws (tyrannosaurs have only two limbs with claws). In fact, it is believed that this is a rudiment, but this lizard clearly helped itself with them to get rid of the carcass of another lizard, supporting it. He, in turn, seemed to me ugly, somehow bony. Part of its intestines dangled from the huge maw of the Tyrannosaurus Rex. I squatted down literally a meter from the mouth of the lizard and began to observe what was happening. He did not pay any attention to me, even when I grabbed the bitten off leg of his victim (it looked like a chicken, but a hundred times larger) and threw it aside. The lizard, again not paying attention to me, raised his head and went for this delicacy. His movements seemed to be difficult for him, and all the muscles of the back of the body simply rolled from the tension, so that there was a feeling of monstrous power. Having gone halfway, the lizard stopped and, looking back, looked at the carcass. He began to return to her. I had already decided to feed him with my hands, but then some kind of siren sounded. Quickly realizing what it was outside the window in the physical world, I immediately plunged headlong into the water in order to get rid of the sound through the programming property of space. In the water, he really became quieter, but he was still there. Watching the pebbles at the bottom in the clear water, I plugged my ears with my fingers. The sound became even quieter. With the tension of the brain, I again increased the vibrations, which caused a noise, which I began to listen to. Siren is gone. I stood up again, pulled my fingers out of my ears, and then it dawned on me that it was a car alarm. "What if it's from my car?" I thought. Cursing everything in the world, he remembered the body in order to return to it. As soon as I felt it, I remembered that the car had been in the car service for several days ... I heard the sound of the siren again, but it was not my car, so it did not make sense to stop the phase. I tried to get into it again, but the howl of the siren did not stop, so all my attempts to return were in vain.

Very important tips

Procedure

So, dear friend, you have decided to change your world, to know its true breadth and possibilities. To do this, you need to understand the procedure. I must say right away that I will not offer you anything very complicated and dreary. Everything is quite simple, especially if done correctly and verbatim.

First, you must start trying to leave the body with your consciousness only with the help of indirect techniques. Focus all your first efforts on describing them and push through until you succeed. Never try direct techniques. Secondly, as soon as you begin to get out of the body, immediately study the deepening and retention of the phase. You only need a few experiences to master these techniques. Thirdly, having learned to go deep and stay in the phase, master the technique of moving and finding objects. This may take a little longer than deepening and holding.

Fourthly, having mastered all the necessary skills, you can draw up an arbitrary plan of action, based on the applied meaning of the phenomenon, and implement it.

Fifth, when the entrance to the phase becomes stable, sometimes (at least 2 times a week) you can start trying direct techniques as well. But do it in such a way that they do not intersect with indirect techniques, that is, they are not performed on the same day. Of course, the described procedure is aimed at achieving a high skill, which is possible only with steady practice and application of the phenomenon. But the emotional return will come much faster. If you have never had a phase experience before, even the first clumsy experience will be the starting point of your development, hitting your consciousness at its very foundation.

Main mistake

If you turn off the path that I am telling you about, then you will either completely lose experience, or it will be very rare. I often have to struggle with one very strange phenomenon of the human psyche: to act on my own in an area in which there is no knowledge. It seems that he checked everything, described everything exactly, you know for sure that it will work. But, when you start to communicate with the next practitioner, it suddenly turns out that all this does not work. At least that's what they tell you. But when a person begins to tell you what and how he did, you literally from the very first words hear about what he asked dozens of times not to do. It turns out that everything is done exactly the opposite. And if the right direction appears, then everything is done by half, by a third, in a different way, the most fundamental things are not completed somewhere. Of course, this is not always the case, but only in cases where a person has problems with practice. If she is not there, he did everything as he was asked . From you, dear friend, I only ask you to follow the instructions verbatim. You are guaranteed to get results. The more correctly you do everything, the faster everything will turn out. Often people get it on the first try.

But let's dwell on the most important mistake in detail. I have repeatedly noted that the practice should be started exclusively with indirect techniques, that is, actions carried out against the backdrop of awakening. I have taught this phenomenon to thousands of people personally and countless numbers through books. And I'm not just saying that this is where you need to start. This is the simplest and most effective. But every second person has an excessive urge to ignore my arguments and start with the most difficult - direct techniques performed without sleep. I am usually told that these techniques are better controlled. Yes, better. But therein lies the problem. That is why techniques do not work for beginners, because they control them. From the section of direct techniques, you will understand that, on the contrary, you need to let go of them, deliberately losing control over them and your consciousness for a while. And this is much more difficult than waking up and getting into the phase in a few seconds.

Outwardly, direct techniques seem to be preferable, and this in itself pushes people to them immediately, although indirect techniques must be well mastered first. Dude, you'll probably have that desire too. But remember in advance one simple thing: indirect techniques work for everyone, and direct ones are difficult even for many experienced ones. What can we say about a beginner who does not yet know the phenomenon from the inside? Starting with direct techniques is like going to the gym for the first time in your life and immediately trying to fully squeeze 200kg. No sober person would do that. This is just unreal. You need to train for a certain time, for which start with small weights. But if the weight on the bar is obvious to the human mind, then the fact that straight techniques are a very close equivalent of the same 200 kg becomes apparent only after months of wasted time and an incredible amount of effort. But everything can happen in just a couple of days ...

Yes, certain individuals have a predisposition towards direct techniques, especially women. But when I talk about it, almost everyone starts to think that this is just about them. Forget about it. First, understand what this phenomenon is through actions against the background of awakening, and only then begin experiments with direct techniques. Moreover, many may think that if they try both direct and indirect techniques at the same time, they will get both a guaranteed practice on the background of awakenings and a likely practice of direct techniques before bedtime, for example. I'll disappoint you right now. You are not a bottomless barrel of emotions and forces. If you are exhausted in the evening on direct techniques, then you will not have enough emotions and strength to competently and effectively do something upon awakening. Having a huge base of observations, I can unequivocally state that this approach reduces the probability of a successful experience by 50-80%. Even more ridiculous is the situation when a person, making some mistakes, failed with indirect techniques, working on them, let's say, for several weeks. I emphasize that this is possible only with gross errors and misunderstandings. So, having stumbled on the easiest, he decides to switch to direct techniques - the most difficult. Where is the logic? If you can't do the simplest thing, what if you can do the most difficult one? Is it so? Just the opposite! If you can't pull the consciousness out of the body on the background of awakening, then the only thing you can still think about is awareness in a dream, but certainly not about direct techniques.

So do not engage in nonsense, but first put all your efforts into actions against the backdrop of awakening - universal indirect techniques. (Sadly, even after such an emphasis, a significant part of readers will still spit on it and begin to suffer with direct techniques ...)

Partial execution of techniques

Another common problem is the incomplete execution of techniques. This affects no less than 75% of practitioners who study using my technologies. Curiously, 75% of them do it intentionally. Friend, later you will see that you don't have to do anything supernatural to reach the phase state. This is a simple algorithm of actions against the background of awakening, if we talk about indirect techniques. And all you need to do is complete it. And do exactly as written. I will give a couple of examples of partial implementation of techniques. Let's say that cycling indirect techniques - an effective universal technology for entering the phase - implies the execution upon awakening of at least 4 cycles of techniques for a total of 9-15 seconds each, if the techniques do not work. For some reason, many people think that the minimum threshold of 4 cycles is nothing more than words. And they do 1-2 cycles... Somehow, at a seminar, two men of approximately the same age (about 45 years old) were sitting side by side. This was the second lesson, and they told what and how they did. The first one said that he did 2 cycles in one attempt, but since nothing worked, he decided not to do more, although I spoke about 4 cycles the day before. I said many times ... The second man also did 2 cycles, and nothing worked for him either. But, as I said, he began to do the 3rd cycle, then the 4th - and some technique "shot" on him, and he was able to get out of the body. But if he had acted like his neighbor, then he would not have succeeded either ... I remember this example well only because the two people sitting next to each other sharply contrasted in their approach to what they were told about.

Also, very often people forget with indirect techniques to first try to separate, and then do cycles. In direct techniques, people forget about the floating state of consciousness, although without it it is generally useless to wait for something, which I also always note first of all. Sometimes the reason for partial fulfillment is not the psychology of a person, but the fact that he cannot fulfill the right thing. For example, with indirect techniques, it is important to wake up without moving, and for many this is not so easy. But you just need to practice. Moreover, at the same time, do not forget: if you woke up on the move, then you still need to do it. Yes, the chances are less, but they are still high. In general, one can endlessly enumerate all sorts of imperfections in techniques. I just wanted to tell you, friend, try to do everything completely. After all, every word of mine in the technical sections is carved by years of teaching, and it weighs much more than it might seem.

You see, picking up this book, you can mistakenly take it as another work on some occult or esoteric practices, where usually everything is given approximately, as if most of the details were left to your own discretion. Do not, under any circumstances, take this approach with respect to this book. Everything is already known, and there is no reason to shroud this practice in a fog of mystery. You have clear instructions. Just do it.

Confidence

At almost every seminar I have to admire the same funny situation. A confused person comes to the second or third lesson and tells his story. Suppose he suddenly woke up in the morning in full consciousness and began to try to get out of the body. Did not work out. Then he tries to apply techniques. Nothing works. Then he frustratedly spits on the whole thing, sends it to hell and decides to continue sleeping. But then he gradually notices that he is no longer in the position in which he woke up. That is, for example, he woke up on his back and did techniques in this position. But after a minute it turns out that he is lying on his stomach! However, he definitely did not move physically. What does it mean?

Buddy, if you doubt whether you will succeed or not, then even if you are in the phase, you will not be able to just stand up, which was what you should have done in such a situation. Any doubt will keep you in the body, pin to it.

And vice versa, in most cases, especially in relation to indirect techniques, it is enough just to be confident, completely convinced that you will now take it and do it! I'm not kidding or exaggerating. It really is. Sometimes it's enough just to want, be sure and act. For several months, I spent every seminar doing research on the effect of confidence on performance. It turned out that 90% of those who get the result do everything confidently, knowing that now or in another attempt they will do it. It also turned out that 90% of those who could not do anything made their attempts uncertainly, without faith in themselves and that they could do it. Draw your own conclusions, my friend. In this book you will find a lot of experiences, not only mine, but also other practitioners. It will give you confidence - and you will do it.

Aspiration

It may seem ridiculous to you to compare such a powerful practice to a barbell (see above), but still, techniques are more related to sports than you might think. Here's another example: the best football forward has the main quality - the mood for a goal, for a shot on goal. When you make attempts to get out of the body, your actions should be very close to this approach. I mean, my friend, situations where you cannot stop there, you always have to literally push yourself further and further. You must understand that luck is in your hands, and not in the fact that someone will do everything for you. You must have a kind of stable vector of efforts directed only at one goal - into the phase!

What it means: you must use every opportunity during the action to get more and more with it. For example, if something suddenly starts to work with indirect techniques, you must use it to the end, try to realize all the chances. It would seem that this is natural and understandable, but many stop at the right moment and begin to observe what will happen next, or move on to another action without realizing the available chance. This should not be. You can't turn to the side. Only forward.

Motivation

If you have already encountered an out-of-body phenomenon, a phase, then you already know how good it is, and you are unlikely to
whether additional motivation will be needed, other than the desire to do it again. But if you have no experience, then you, my friend, must first either delve into the incredible essence of the phenomenon, or read more about its applied significance. If you do it out of curiosity - just try it and see what happens - you may not succeed. You must really want it. When this desire is sharp and deep, everything will turn out much better for you. Moreover, this will often happen even without your will - that's how powerful the power of intention and desire is!

Timing and efficiency

Buddy, you may be very surprised, but I always cut off people who, on emotions, declare that everything is so cool that they are ready to spend at least a month, at least six months, on the first experience in order to experience it at least once. I'm sorry because with the right actions you need only a few attempts, which you can do in one day ...

Yes, it's not as easy as imagining something or imagining how to take a pill or smoke weed. This requires action and effort. Sometimes a lot of tries. But, having done everything right, you will get the result quickly enough. Remember this simple thing: if you do indirect techniques every week for a week and nothing works out for you, you are doing something wrong. You need to read more carefully about the techniques and try to find errors. Believe me, you will have a huge number of mistakes, even when you manage to get into the phase. On average, a beginner makes up to 7-10 typical mistakes each time in his first attempts ... So read carefully and analyze each of your actions.

In general, to get the effect due to indirect techniques, you need about 5 attempts in the normal case and up to 20 attempts with gross errors. If we talk about lucid dreaming, it can take from 1 to 20 days. If you have mastered indirect techniques, then after another 5-30 attempts, direct techniques will begin to work, that is, carried out without prior sleep. However, the latter are much more difficult to master. They may not be available at all if you do not understand the essence of the floating state of consciousness. The main thing is to make regular attempts. The question is only in them and their quality. There will be attempts - there will be a result. Everything is simple, as always.

The golden ratio of practice and ordinary life

I am often asked the same question: since the world of the phase is so beautiful and has such crazy possibilities, does it make you want to stay there or just ignore real life? I always answer this in the same way: this practice itself will not be so beautiful if you have problems in your life; these two worlds mutually adorn each other; when things are going well here and there, then the effect is multiplied many times over. It really is. Whether you like it or not, there is still reality. You spend most of your life in it, and you should not spoil it. Few people know that such words are far from simple reflection. This is an experience. Indeed, some time ago, back in my youth, when faced with the phenomenon of a phase, I allowed very large excesses. My daily life really collapsed in all possible forms. And the further, the less I wanted to return to it. The accumulated problems deprived me of peace, and this greatly affected my general well-being. At some critical moment, the phase stopped saving, and I changed my life. I began to pay attention to the physical world, to well-being in it, using the possibilities of the phase itself for this ...

Gradually I became successful both here and there. And these two worlds really began to decorate each other, making me doubly, no, triple happier. Having experienced all this on myself, I now first of all ask you, my friend, to approach this phenomenon from exactly the same position. And you will be happy. You must be a master out of the body, you must be beautiful, healthy and agile with your physical body, you must be successful in your affairs. Happiness is in your hands. And it is multifaceted. It makes no sense to deal with only one facet of this diamond. Well, don't forget that the phase can help you in all this. Take a quick look at the applied side of the phenomenon - and you will easily understand it.

Example from practice:

August, 2008
Waking up at about eight in the morning, took a cold shower, but still could not tune in to work. Decided to go back to sleep. Given that this is a good time to try to get into the phase, I decided to try to do something. To anything but a phantom rocking, the soul did not lie. Not particularly hoping to get an effect, monotonously and routinely began to try to swing the brush with a "boat". She, in turn, quickly succumbed to the movement, although initially the amplitude was very small.
Almost already falling asleep, I noticed that the amplitude increased sharply, and the arm began to literally twist. I decided to monitor the situation more closely and twisted my arm more and more in one direction or the other. At some point, the arm twisted almost 360 °. Then it dawned on me that the perception of the whole body had changed significantly. Clearly, something was happening. Tried to roll out. It did not work out, but on the background of the attempt, vibrations arose. This was the signal to try to roll out even more actively. I tried it and it worked. With difficulty, viscous, but gone. He rolled out in his room,

but the condition was unstable: there were no clear sensations and he was drawn back to the body. He began to randomly feel everything. Gradually, the thrust into the body disappeared, and after 5-10 seconds vision began to appear, which I began to use to deepen my gaze. This turned out to be the decisive move. The phase has become hyper-realistic. I immediately remembered what I should have tried to do in this phase, and started from the main point - experiments with movement. I wanted to check once again how difficult it is to move in space using the door technique. First, closed the door. I focused on the fact that behind it is the audience in which I conduct classes. He opened the door, went into the auditorium and closed the door again. Now I focused on the fact that instead of my room, behind the door is a gym where I work out. Opened - I see the hall. He immediately closed the door and opened it again - still a hall. He walked in and closed the door behind him. He focused his attention on the fact that there is open space behind the door. He opened the door, and behind it was a corridor, which should be in reality if you are in the hall. He closed it and focused his attention even more strongly on the space behind the door. He began to open the door, but it was as if something was holding it from the other side. I had to use force to start to open slightly, and then the movement went easily. At that moment, I noticed that the space began to blur, but I managed to concentrate and, with the help of brain tension, restored realism. Behind the door was open space. I stood on the threshold of the hall, and literally a step away from me there was an endless space without top and bottom. Breathed freely. An icy cold blew from the door. Experience has shown that by this method it is still more difficult to get anywhere except from room to room; probably, this happens only because of the internal blocks of human consciousness. While I stood and analyzed what was happening, I began to be sucked into a stencil. The only thing that could be used at that very moment was to grab onto the door handles, which I did, and almost unconsciously, on the machine. I feel like I'm in my body. But the hand clearly continues to hold the door handle. I began to rotate the phantom arm in all planes and soon felt that I could separate. He rolled out easily and was back in his room. He quickly brought the state to hyper-realism by looking, mixed with groping, and, feeling that he had almost completed the obligatory work, he gave free rein to his inner desire to meet the girl A. (I had not seen her for a long time, but I continued to have certain feelings for her). I went to the bathroom door and opened it without a moment's hesitation, knowing that I would find her there. And so it happened. I opened the door and saw that behind it was the room of my apartment, where I used to live and where I once met this girl. Of course, I expected to see her naked right in the bath, but it was not bad anyway ... She sat on the couch and looked towards the window. I felt that she understood that I was there. He walked over and sat on the floor across from her. He began to touch her, stroke her. In view of the hyper-realism, the sensations were incredibly vivid and amazing. Simply stroking her skirt and jacket was an incredible experience, just like it used to be in reality. It was very pleasant to feel her tender and warm body under her clothes, thin knees and stockings. I reached out to her head, and when I began to remove the hair from her face, she turned in my direction and smiled. In response to the look of those same eyes and that same smile, there was nothing left to do but smile back. At the same time, he continued to run his hands over her face, head and body to hold her. Her eyes were sad, and her smile - as if through tears. But with all this, her look was more open and sincere than when all this happened in reality. A. also started touching my face and hands. Then she began to ask how I was doing and what I was doing. Realizing that this communication was only a formality, which was secondary in the phase, I answered in monosyllables, enjoying the very fact that I was next to the girl, I could touch her, see her eyes and hear a painfully familiar voice. Surprisingly, I was not overcome by unbridled sexual instincts, which usually arise when communicating with the opposite sex in the phase. After staying with her for some more time, I decided that it was time to end the date, as I could see her another time. It was still necessary to try many times to enter the body and leave it to practice this skill, which was planned in the original plan of action. Deliberately returned to the body and immediately began to try to get out of it. It was easy to roll out. Came back and rolled out again. However, after the next return, the connection with reality increased greatly, and I had to make a fair amount of effort to literally get out of the body. For this, it was also necessary to apply force falling asleep.

Once again in the middle of the room, I clearly understood that it was better not to return to the body yet. But deliberately, without even fixing the phase with a deepening, he rushed back anyway to find out the limit of his own capabilities and hone his exit skill even more. Once in the stencil, at first I could barely move, but then a wave of awakening swept over me. Switched to force sleep and then observation of images, since the first did not work. The images did not appear. I again began to try to separate, although there was a complete sense of the final awakening. He began to try to push his arms along the body and pull them back. After a few seconds, a phantom movement arose, and consciousness immediately went a little deeper from the outside world. I concentrated even more on the movement, and it went even more. I started trying to get up. It went, but very viscous. The body seemed to weigh several times more. With any relaxation, I was immediately chained back to the stencil. At some point, I managed to separate completely and find myself near the bed. I tried to randomly use all possible deepening techniques, but nothing helped, and I returned to the body. Couldn't get out of it anymore.

Chapter Two

The exit of consciousness from the body

It is time to learn in practice what Higher Yoga is. From this moment on, all empty talk ends, and we begin to open the door to a parallel world. Once again, dear friend, all the technical sections and information in this book are not approximate descriptions of supposed actions, but specific instructions with mandatory verbatim execution. This is especially true in this part of the book. Do not blame the technique and incompetence of the author if you do everything carelessly and unpedantically. It's unlikely that you'll be able to do anything. If it says here that something needs to be done, then it is exactly what it is. If it is said that it is not necessary to do something, then this is not said for the red word, but for your own good, no matter how it seems to you. Moreover, everything is described literally, and there is no need to interpret anything in your own way. Understand, the author did not come up with all this two months ago, but worked out for ten years on thousands of people and certainly knows well what you should and should not do.

Indirect technique

Indirect techniques are actions for entering the phase state, carried out against the background of awakening. This is where any practitioner should start. If you, dear friend, ignore this fact, you are unlikely to succeed at all. Or rather, you won't succeed at all if, for example, you start your journey with direct techniques, when all actions are carried out without prior sleep.

Many mistakenly believe that indirect techniques work like a pill - easy and simple the first time. Despite the fact that the technologies described in this book are an order of magnitude superior to any other in their effectiveness, some effort on your part is still needed. For some, this clarification is irrelevant, since everything will turn out very easily, but for someone it can be very useful, because it will take about 10 attempts.

Try to understand the important things first:

• Everything will work for sure if you follow the steps in sequence, as described in the book.

• With indirect techniques, everything depends only on the number of attempts.

It has already been noted that in most cases only a few full attempts are enough when waking up without movement. Even if it takes longer than usual to achieve the result, this does not mean that the techniques are not suitable for you. This simply cannot be - and this must also be clearly understood. It's all about mistakes. Attempts are important in many ways not only to achieve the final result, but also for the very process of achieving it. Making attempts, the practitioner independently finds answers to questions. Much is simply impossible to put into words. Something is bound to be missed. During conscious attempts to get into the phase, a person himself must draw conclusions, which, of course, will be useful and will speed up the results. There should be more specifics in your actions. First, the most suitable techniques are studied and selected. At the same time, the goal is to wake up consciously and without movement. Trying to do cycles of indirect techniques at this moment every day is the next goal. With such clear-cut actions, in no case should you defocus your attention and scatter emotions on adjacent actions, for example, on direct techniques for entering the phase or something else. All efforts are only for the most important thing.

Although it often takes only one or two days, in any case it is a matter of a maximum of weeks, and not months or even several years, as previously thought. You just need to stubbornly achieve your goal - step by step, clearly, meticulously. However, if there is no effect after 10-20 days, then it is worth leaving the practice for a week and taking a break from it, so that later you can start over with renewed vigor. Curiously, it is during such a break that spontaneous falling into the phase occurs. When, after a break, you start the practice again, carefully study the whole theory in order to understand your mistakes. Once again, I emphasize: the problem is always in them, and not in the techniques themselves. Having done a huge number of workshops, and having a crazy amount of observations, I can swear by the holiest thing in my life that this is the only way.

Techniques

There are a huge number of techniques, but I'm not going to scatter your attention on what doesn't work very well. Below are only those techniques that most clearly manifest themselves in practice, which was unambiguously proven at the same seminars.

Buddy, you do not need to strive to understand all the techniques and manage all of them - from the entire list you need to choose 3-4 most suitable ones. You should not take on some techniques just because they seem interesting, or because someone has written or talked a lot about them. You need to be based solely on what suits you specifically. Of all the main indirect techniques listed above, only 95% of students get the tension of the brain easily and quickly. All other techniques succeed only 25-50% of practitioners on the first training attempt. However, after several trainings, at least 75% of students master each technique. It is through such training that you must discover what is yours and what is not. Although, you know, at the moment of direct practice, what you least expected often works.

The development of techniques, preliminary training with them is carried out in such a way that for at least three days you should experiment with each of them for 2-10 minutes during the daytime. Only such training will allow you to accurately determine which of the techniques is right for you. In addition, another problem is solved in this way: during the choice of techniques, the best memorization and assimilation of the techniques themselves occurs, which definitely has a positive effect on their application at the right time.

In any case, everyone notes for himself a certain set of techniques that he does better than others. There should be at least three of them, and even better - four or five, so that there is always a choice for combinations. Moreover, all non-working techniques still need to be kept in mind and sometimes tried to apply. You never know what your body is capable of in different attempts. At the same time, do not forget that the techniques you finally choose should be diverse, affecting different types of perception: visual, sound, kinesthetic, vestibular.

Force falling asleep

Highest application recommendation. Waking up without movement and without opening the eyelids, you need to portray a quick forced falling asleep for 5-10 seconds. During this process, it is necessary to have an attitude that there will be no final falling asleep, but a sharp return to consciousness, after which an attempt to separate will follow. As a rule, after such a trick with the brain, the state of consciousness changes dramatically and strong vibrations can occur on the "emergence" from pseudo-sleep, or it will be easy to separate, or other techniques begin to work well. This forced falling asleep is, in fact, a trick of the brain. The brain reflexively reacts to the actions of a person and quickly puts him into a sleepy state, which is easy to use to enter the phase. This technique is especially effective if applied when waking up too abruptly or after an inadvertent physical movement was made during awakening (opened eyes, turned around, scratched). In such cases, always remember this magical technique, which creates a kind of rollback to a deeper state.

Whatever you think, power falling asleep is very simple. You need to turn off the internal dialogue, move away from external stimuli and just want to quickly fall asleep, but after a few seconds you will come to your senses again. To understand how this is done, it is enough to remember how falling asleep occurred against the background of severe fatigue or a long lack of sleep and when you urgently needed to fall asleep. The most common mistake is that people actually fall asleep by doing the technique too actively and simply forgetting that there is always the possibility of unplanned falling asleep for real.

And I will also give you one great piece of advice: you can use force falling asleep in parallel with any other techniques, which increases their effectiveness many times over. For example, it happens that you wake up, you try a phantom rocking, but it does not happen -

there is not even a hint. You start pretending to fall asleep and then again you try to make a phantom rocking - and it immediately appears! Naturally, if you know what it is and have previously worked in training. By the way, you can also work out in power falling asleep. Of course, the desired state will not arise, and you are unlikely to fall asleep during daily workouts, but you will remember what and how you did, so that at the right time it can only be reproduced.

Phantom sway

Highest application recommendation. Waking up without movement and without opening the eyelids, within 3-5 seconds you need to try to phantom swing any part of the body. If nothing swings during this time, the technique needs to be changed. If even a slight swaying is felt, then you need to continue, striving for only one; maximize the range of motion. This must be done very aggressively and persistently. Once the amplitude is close to 10 cm or more, which may take only a few seconds, the following situations are possible:
• an attempt to separate from the body;
• the swinging part of the body begins to move freely, and, starting from it, you can calmly separate, literally stand up;
• there are strong vibrations against which you can try to separate;
• there is a noise to which it is necessary to listen, that too can lead to a phase;
• you instantly and involuntarily find yourself in some place in the phase.
It makes sense to separately focus on the very concept of phantom swaying, since about half of the students

initially misunderstand them. Buddy, this is not some imaginary movement of some phantom body. Initially, a person tries to make a movement with a real hand, simply without straining the muscles. That is, there is some inner desire to make a movement without it in the physical plane. When the sensation arises, it is not much different from the real, and it is often accompanied by sensations of viscosity and resistance. As a rule, the movement is initially low-amplitude, in the range of only a centimeter or even a millimeter, but with due effort, the amplitude increases and becomes larger and larger each time. You only need to swing the part of the body more and more, pull it in one direction or the other.

One of the signs of the correct execution of the phantom swing: doubt whether you are doing this with a physical hand? Remember, initially you begin to swing your physical hand (feeling it), without imagining anything at all. In turn, if the hand always swings easily and widely, even during daytime training, then this is a sign of a gross mistake - imagining the movement with a figurative hand. This is a completely different technique - a visual movement.

It also does not matter in which part of the body the phantom movement is called. You can move at least with your whole body, at least with one finger. Also, the frequency of movement does not matter. The key is amplitude. In order to practice performing phantom swings, you should lie down with your eyes closed for several minutes, relax your hand. Then, for 2-3 minutes, without straining the physical muscles, you need to try to make the following movements with it: up and down, left and right, swinging the boat, clenching and unclenching the fist, etc.

Keep in mind that at first no sensations arise, but gradually, in the course of performing some exercises, a subtle movement begins to be felt. Often in the initial stages, a person wants to open his eyes and see if he is actually making a movement or not - this is such a plausible feeling. By the way, with indirect techniques, upon awakening, you should immediately try to swing something for 3-5 seconds without first relaxing.

Observation of images

Highest application recommendation. Waking up without movement and without opening the eyelids, for 3-5 seconds you need to peer into the space in front of your eyes, trying to see any images, pictures, etc. in it. If there is nothing, the technique should be changed. If something appears, you need to peer into these images further. At the same time, they will quickly become more realistic, as if absorbing you. In no case should you consider the details of the image, otherwise it will disappear or change. Everything should be viewed in a panoramic way, entirely, including the whole picture in the review of attention at once, and not particulars. You need to observe the images as long as there is a dynamics of increasing their quality and realism. As a result, two variants of the development of events are possible: a person will find himself in an observable image, in fact, in a phase, or the image will become absolutely real, after which it will only be necessary to immediately separate from the body. The latter is preferable as it gives you more control over your actions and reduces the chances of falling asleep during the attempt.

To practice with images, you need to lie in the dark with your eyes closed for several minutes to peer into the void in front of you and catch any specific images that can start with simple, meaningless points and gradually turn into complete pictures, actions, plots. As a result, one can easily learn how to create images and then apply them very effectively against the backdrop of awakening. Often the mistake is that the practitioner tries to create an image when one should simply try to see it. It has to come up on its own, buddy.

Hand visualization

Highest application recommendation. Waking up without moving and without opening your eyelids, for 3-5 seconds you need to try to see your hands in front of you from a distance of 5-20 cm, just above eye level. You need to do this with a desire, by all means, as if there really are hands there, but for some reason they are not felt and they are not visible. If nothing happens during this time, the technique changes to another. If hands begin to appear, they will simply be felt before the eyes, or both at the same time, then you need to stop at the technique until these sensations become absolutely vivid. As soon as the hands are visible in the same way as if they were usually looked at, then it remains just to stand up. You can also get up if the hands are not visible, but they are well felt before the eyes, and not where they should lie. In turn, where they should lie, they should not be felt at all. It is worth noting that you need to try not only to see the hands, but also to feel them in front of you. Don't do this technique sluggishly and statically. On the contrary, in all moments show maximum activity, an all-consuming desire. For example, keep your hands in front of you, not just imagining, but twist them, clench them into fists, three against each other, etc., etc. Naturally, trying to feel and see it.

It is very easy to train in this technique, for example, during the day. Of course, as with other trainings of techniques, it will not work to the end, and you will not get into the phase, but then you will be able to work out the action itself, the power of intention with it, which cannot but affect the practice itself at the right moment, about which will be discussed a little later.

Rotation

Highest application recommendation. Waking up without movement and without opening the eyelids, within 3-5 seconds you need to mentally begin to rotate around its axis. Unlike phantom swings, here it is necessary to represent the movement, and as reliably as possible. If no unusual sensations arise, the technique must be changed. If, however, vibrations occur during the rotation, or suddenly the rotation becomes sensationally unimaginable, but real, you need to continue to perform it further until the dynamics are observed. There are several options for the development of further events:

• you can try to separate immediately;

• representation of rotation is replaced by a real feeling, and to enter the phase it remains just to move to the side;

• there are strong vibrations, strong noise, against which;

• you can separate from the body or jump to the appropriate techniques;

• during rotation, it can simply be thrown out of the body, or a person can suddenly find himself in some space in the phase.

As with other techniques, in order to separately practice rotation, you need to lie with your eyes closed for several minutes to imagine the rotation of the body around its axis. There is no need to focus on the visual consequences of rotation and on the detailed sensations of the body. The most important thing is vestibular sensations from internal turns. As a rule, many initially have difficulties with a full turn. Someone can turn only a quarter, someone - half. However, with this you just need to practice a little longer - and everything will start to work out.

Eavesdropping

Waking up without movement and without opening the eyelids, within 3-5 seconds you need to try to hear the noise in your head. If it was not there during this time, you need to change the technique. If there is noise or buzz, hum, roar, hiss, whistle, ringing, melody, you need to start listening to this sound, trying to better recognize it. The volume will definitely increase. You need to listen until there is some dynamics in the increase in sound. As soon as it stops or the sound becomes loud enough, you can try to separate from the body. Sometimes noise simply throws a person out of phase while listening. In the final stage, the noise can be so strong that it can only be compared with the roar of a jet engine, located very close by. This often frightens beginners, and many have encountered this phenomenon even without phase practices.

Listening is an attempt to carefully hear the sound, all its tones and frequencies. There is another version of force listening, when you just want to increase the noise, while making internal intuitive efforts, which, as a rule, are correct. If the noise at this time begins to increase, then the consequences will be the same as with normal listening. If you want to practice listening, you need to lie in silence with your eyes closed and try to listen "inside the head." Usually, within a few minutes, these attempts are crowned with success, and the person begins to hear the noise. Everyone is capable of hearing such noise, you just need to be able to tune in to it. Either way, it only takes a couple of workouts to get it right.

Brain tension

Waking up without movement and without opening the eyelids, you need to do two or three compressions, tensions of the brain. If nothing happens, the technique needs to be changed. If vibrations arise, they should be strengthened and moved through the body by the same tension of the brain. The stronger the vibrations, the more likely it will be to separate or spontaneously eject from the body. In addition, noise may occur, which can also be exploited by listening.

Feelings of vibration cannot be confused with anything. If a person doubts whether he experienced them or not, then most likely he did not experience them. In perception, they are similar to a strong current passing through the body and not causing pain, to a strong numbness of the whole body at once, to its strong compression, or to all of this at the same time. In general, you will immediately understand when you encounter this.

To train with brain tension, you need to lie down with your eyes closed and try to strain your brain without thinking that this is impossible. Tension should be done spasmodic and rhythmic. Sometimes you can delay the voltage in the power phase. You can strain both the whole brain and its individual parts. In the process, there is a feeling of pressure or even real tension in the head, oddly enough, my friend. Usually this exercise is easy for almost everyone from the very first minutes. During training, you need to remember well how this tension is caused, so that you can reproduce it later on waking up. Very often, when performing this technique, the following mistake is made: instead of trying to strain something inside the head, they begin to strain the muscles of the face and neck. This should not be done otherwise there will be no result at the right time. Moreover, it will bring down the whole state, because the physical body should in no case participate in the process.

Dot on the forehead

Waking up without movement and without opening the eyelids, within 3-5 seconds, you need to reduce the focus of vision towards a point in the middle of the forehead. If nothing happens, the technique changes. If vibrations arise, then with the help of concentration on a point or even simultaneous tension of the brain, they can be strengthened, and then separated. It is also possible that there will be noise that you can listen to.
It is worth noting separately that this technique is especially good in conjunction with brain tension. They seem to reinforce each other. Moreover, as in the case of force falling asleep, rolling the eyes to a point in the forehead significantly enhances any parallel technique. This is probably due to the fact that when falling asleep we always roll our eyes up a little, although you might not notice this. That is, the reflex is also triggered here.
It is important to note: you do not need to roll your eyes with effort. It should be as natural as possible. If

something powerful appears, it will have the opposite effect - the entire pre-phase state will be lost.

Motion representation

Waking up without movement and without opening your eyelids, for 5-10 seconds, concentrate on any of the following actions: rocking, walking, running, somersaulting, tug of war, swimming, rotating your arms, etc. You just need to try to imagine the actions as you can more realistic, all the time. If nothing happens, the technique changes. The execution of a technique can be considered successful if the presented movements become the main ones in the sensation, which, as a rule, is accompanied by a movement to some place in the phase. If such a movement does not automatically occur, you can try to separate as soon as you understand that the idea has been replaced by a completely real (I emphasize) sensation. As strange as it may seem, this is actually how it happens. Also, do not forget to pre-train with these ideas during the day for at least a few minutes, which will significantly increase the effectiveness of the technique at the right time.

Separation Techniques

Dear friend, always remember that in one third of successful cases of indirect entry into the phase upon awakening, it is not necessary to perform any of the specific techniques that we have just discussed. It is possible to separate immediately. This is unshakably proven in the statistics of the results of the seminars and is obvious when conducting independent experiments. But misunderstanding separation techniques leads to negative consequences. It happens that even if a person is in a phase state, he still cannot separate. Therefore, it is very important to understand what separation techniques are, because sometimes mastering them plays a key role in the whole practice, which is understandable.

Often it is enough to think about separation, how it immediately happens on its own. But this is not always the case, so there are a number of auxiliary techniques. The most important of them are rolling out, getting up, getting out and taking off. At the same time, all separation techniques are united by one common point: you can't imagine anything, but you need to try to make a movement with your own body without straining your muscles. This manifests itself literally in the same way as if a similar movement was made for real. If nothing happens after a few seconds of trying, it means that right now it does not work. If it works, it will be immediately noticeable. Moreover, often people are so unprepared for the reality of sensations that they think that they are making a movement physically, because of which they return back to the body, and only later, by indirect signs, do they understand what happened to them.

It happens that the separation has passed, but not completely or with some effort and hard. This, however, is a signal that everything is being done correctly and that you just need to add strength and aggression in order to completely separate. For example, if some movement started and stopped after some progress, you need to go back and move in the same direction again with greater intensity. You can also randomly alternate these techniques.

To practice separation techniques, you just need to lie down and, with your eyes closed, try to perform them all in turn for several minutes. Most likely, everything is done correctly if, during the attempt to separate, no muscles are twitching or tensing, and even more so, there is no physical movement, but there is a strong, almost physically tangible internal desire to make a movement. In this case, of course, in reality, no movement occurs, and the person simply lies in place. Immediately upon awakening, such actions will often lead to easy entry into phase space. So it's really a key skill.

getting up

You just need to try to get out of bed without straining your muscles. This should be done in the way that seems most convenient at a particular moment. Don't overthink it, just try to do it. Imagine nothing, as in other techniques.

rolling out

Try to roll, without straining your muscles, to the edge of the bed, off it, or towards the wall. You don't have to think about falling or how it should feel in detail. You just need to roll without straining your muscles. Try to do it.

crawling out

Here you need to try to literally get out of your body without straining your muscles. As a rule, this technique spontaneously comes to mind when there is only a partial separation using other techniques or only one part of the body is divided.

Takeoff

You need to try to literally fly up, being parallel to the bed. There is no need to think about how to take off, because intuitively you yourself know what to do, because this is familiar from ordinary dreams. You can also try the same thing, but down - falling through the bed.

When to do indirect techniques

By far the best option for indirect techniques is the delayed method. Its essence is to interrupt sleep in the final stages and then fall asleep, which leads to superficial sleep in the remaining time. That is, such a dream will be accompanied by frequent awakenings, which can be fruitfully used to enter the phase. If you go to bed at 00:00, then you need to set an alarm for 6:00 in the morning. Awakening must be clearly recorded, for which you need to do something for several minutes. For example, read this chapter and determine your actions, go to the toilet, drink juice, etc. After that, you need to go to bed thinking that there will be many awakenings in the next 2-4 hours and each time you will need to make attempts to get into phase. Naturally, if you go to bed earlier, then the alarm clock should also ring exactly after 6 hours - this is the best option for entering the phase. If less time passes, then in the second half the sleep will be deep, if more, then there will be little time left for attempts, and in general, you can simply not fall asleep again. However, the later you go to bed, the shorter this interval should be, given the biorhythms. Of course, we are talking about the case if it is unusual for you. If you tend to wake up too abruptly, after which it is difficult to fall asleep, then getting out of bed after the alarm is not necessary. You can immediately go to bed and catch the next awakenings by thinking carefully about them. The delayed method is best used in cases where it is possible to sleep without restrictions, in any case, without an early rise. Not everyone can afford such a luxury on a daily basis. However, almost everyone has a weekend when you can find time to test this method. If it is possible not to get up early, you must definitely use this time for the phase, since it is many times more effective than other periods of time. Pay close attention to this if you want to get a quick result.

The second most effective period of time useful for experiencing the phase is the usual single morning awakening. As a rule, this occurs against the background of superficial sleep with a rested consciousness. Also, an equally effective period of time for the use of indirect techniques is waking up after a daytime sleep. Maybe it's even better than waking up in the morning. In this case, sleep will also be superficial and short, which will allow the body to rest, and memory and intention can easily be preserved until the moment of awakening. Although most of the spontaneous entrances into the phase occur at night, the night awakenings themselves are the least effective for deliberate practice due to the fact that at night the brain needs a lot of time for normal deep sleep, therefore, against the background of awakening , the consciousness is clouded and the ability to do something is very small. . Even if something turns out, it very often ends with a quick fall asleep. However, this does not mean that practice is not possible at night. It's just that attempts will not be as effective as at other times of the day.

It should also be understood that we wake up every 90 minutes at night anyway, even if we don't remember it, so even for a six-hour sleep, at least four awakenings are guaranteed. When a practitioner knows about this and seeks to capture these moments, he really begins to use them over time.

Conscious awakening

To start performing indirect techniques upon awakening, it is not enough just to know them and wake up. Due to the peculiarities of the human consciousness and its habits, it is difficult, having barely woken up, to immediately recall a specific action. Moreover, here we are talking about the fact that you need to remember the action instantly, and not after lying down for several minutes or even seconds. This is the conscious awakening, without the ability to do without which you will not succeed, my friend, although this is not such a great difficulty, given the ultimate goal. According to my observations, for about a quarter of practitioners this is nothing difficult, but for the rest it can be a small obstacle with which to sometimes tinker. If you belong to the latter, then you just need to understand: nothing is impossible and everything is achieved through persistent attempts and constant training. The reasons for not being able to remember the phase upon awakening are as follows: the lack of the habit of doing something immediately after waking up , desire to sleep further, go to the toilet, drink, start daily activities, etc.
Keep in mind from the very beginning that conscious awakening with the intention of attempting an indirect technique should be the very first, main goal to be achieved at any cost. It is necessary to concentrate on this, because not only the speed of mastering the phase

depends on this moment, but also the very fact of experiencing it in general - in the event that a person has never encountered it. But while you can try all this on pure faith. Here are some helpful technical tips to help you.

Sleep intention

There is a proven scientific fact: in most cases, a person, but waking up, thinks about what he thought about falling asleep. This is especially noticeable if he is worried about some serious life problem. With this problem, he falls asleep and gets up with it. If you deliberately concentrate on waking up before going to bed and trying to get into the phase during it, then this will certainly have an effect. Not necessarily, falling asleep, just think about it. It is enough just to clearly and distinctly fix this desire. You can even say it to yourself or out loud. It helps a lot here to scroll through the mind of the actions that will need to be performed when awakening. If, for example, these are cycles of indirect techniques, then they need to be scrolled through in the mind several times with concentration.

Creating Motivation

As you understand, the greater the intention and desire to get into the phase for the sake of some goal, the faster you can learn to consciously awaken, and the faster the result will be obtained. This is undeniable. Work in this direction. The motivation can be a strong desire to do or experience something in the phase. In general, the very fact of being in this state can play a huge motivating role, but an unprepared person does not know this, and he needs something more understandable. For example, one should immediately realize the applied significance of the phase. For some it will be an opportunity to fly to Mars, for someone to see a dead person, for someone it will be a chance to get some information or influence the course of the disease, etc.

In terms of effectiveness, the best time for a conscious awakening is the moment of "surfacing" from a dream, and not a full normal awakening. This will be the most effective and fruitful effect if you immediately begin to try to separate from the body or perform techniques. As a rule, at this moment a person does not even have time to feel his body. Often this happens against the background of a short-term awareness at the very end of a dream, against the backdrop of a nightmare, pain in a dream, etc. And so, leaving a dream in such a situation, you should immediately try to do something, while you are not yet in the body . This, of course, does not always work out, but consider in advance: if this can be, this should also be used, and with double certainty. When there is regular practice, a reflex should be developed that allows you to perform the planned actions at the moment of awakening, when awareness has not yet come to you. This will allow you to capture the best moments.

Of course, using the phase of absolutely all awakenings for practice is hardly achievable. Therefore, you should not be upset if the necessary awareness upon awakening does not come every time. Normal is at least two or three such awakenings per day, if their total number was two to three times more. This is quite enough for active practice - from two to five phases per week with everyday attempts. But here I want to warn you: don't try too hard. This leads to failure. Let you have only 3-4 attempts in one morning, for example, but they will be of high quality and you will sleep well in front of them. Much worse, if you are exhausted during the night in endless awakenings, you won't get anything because of this, and you won't get enough sleep. Everything should be natural and harmonious.

Cycles of indirect techniques

So, the techniques for creating the phase and the technique of separation in the phase were considered above, the conscious awakening and the time for its best implementation were studied. Now a specific algorithm of actions for indirect techniques will be considered, the implementation of which should lead to the greatest and fastest practical effect.
However, first I will make one more important digression. It is about awakening without moving. Waking up, try not to move in any case, if there is no significant discomfort, which is better to remove and then just do something. If your actions during the cycles of indirect techniques are accompanied by a preliminary slight physical movement, then you will simply have significantly less chances for a result. But, attention, do not make a typical mistake that is very offensive to me personally: if you even move a little, then still make attempts, use all the chances, especially since they are still great. For some reason, most ignore my words about this, and end up with rarer experiences than they could have. Not only that, but what if there is a global problem with awakenings without movement? Some get so stupid that they do nothing all this time ... And instead of everyday attempts, they have one or two a week, although they could have up to 5 a day. So draw your own conclusions. So, the cycles of indirect

techniques are the only universal algorithm for entering the phase (Higher Yoga).

1. Separations (3-5 seconds)

If you remember, in a third of the cases of successful application of indirect techniques, the practitioner does not have to apply the techniques themselves as such, since separation techniques immediately work. This is due to the fact that the first seconds are the most fruitful for the phase. The less time has passed after waking up, the better - this is the main rule. And vice versa, if you lie down and wait for something, then the chances are rapidly melting away. That is why, upon waking up, preferably without movement, immediately begin to quickly sort through the techniques of separation, putting your soul into each of them. For example, rolling out, getting up, taking off. If at least some technique suddenly begins to manifest itself in about 5 seconds, you need to stop at the separation and completely separate at all costs. Sometimes, during separation, there are sensations of ductility, heaviness, a barrier. You don't need to pay attention to this, you should still separate - stubbornly and aggressively, trying to literally get out of yourself, although more often it turns out quite easily.

Trying to separate as soon as you wake up is one of the most important skills to master from the very beginning and never forget about it. Naturally, this makes more sense the longer you wake up without physical movement. If it all started with him, then you'd better skip this point, and instead do a power fall asleep for 5-10 seconds, then proceed again to the separation and then point 2.

2. Cycle of indirect techniques

Nevertheless, in most cases, it is not possible to separate in the first few seconds, so you need to proceed to the next steps. Only now it is necessary to try to apply the phase creation techniques. From the list of indirect techniques, you should have already chosen at least three of the most suitable ones. It is now these techniques that need to be adopted.

To be specific, we'll look at three specific techniques that you should replace with your own techniques when you're trying to do it yourself. Let's say these are the most effective techniques: observation of images, phantom swaying and rotation. After an unsuccessful attempt to separate, you should immediately peer into the emptiness before your eyes. If within 3-5 seconds you notice that you are seeing some pictures of images, then you need to immediately begin to review them without peering into small details, otherwise everything will be lost. In response, the image will quickly become more realistic and colorful, as if absorbing into itself. With luck, you suddenly move into an image or, when it becomes very real, you simply separate from the body. If initially nothing worked for 3-5 seconds, that is, the image did not even appear, you move on to the phantom swing technique. Using the same 3-5 seconds, quickly examine the entire body for the swinging part. Or, this time can be spent trying to swing a certain part of the body, such as a finger, arm or leg. If the effect appears, you must stop on this technique and achieve the maximum amplitude, during which it will either spontaneously eject from the body, or you will be able to separate, or the swinging part will begin to move freely, or vibrations or noise will occur, which can also be used further. If initially nothing swayed in 3-5 seconds, then immediately proceed to rotation, do not stop at this technique.

During the same time (3-5 seconds) try to imagine the rotation. If it turns out and it causes some interesting sensations, you continue to do it further. Once the rotation becomes perceptually real, or unusually easy to do, one can try to separate from the body. If initially nothing happened in 3-5 seconds, you need to do everything all over again, from observing the images. In reality, there may not be three technicians, but more or less. The bottom line is that they need to be changed and that they should be used every time you try. This is because the body often reacts specifically to them. For the same person, the same technique works one day, but not the other, while another one works, which, for example, did not work on the previous day. Therefore, if you perform any one technique, albeit a very good one, often effective, you can lose most of the practice. And this is a gross mistake that almost all practitioners make. Please do not step on the same rake! You will deprive yourself of a large part of the practice. There must be several technicians. One does not work - the other will work, and so every time.

In connection with the execution of techniques, it is very important to note a typical mistake - the relaxed execution of techniques, without the desire to achieve their maximum manifestation. In such cases, people get a manifestation of the technique, but instead of trying to make rapid progress, they do everything calmly and do not strive for anything. But the desire to get into the phase should be clearly expressed. You must understand: if a technique manifests itself during your awakening, then you are already almost in the phase and you only need to strengthen it at all costs. Remember, if upon awakening , some technique immediately manifested itself, and you did not get into the phase, you yourself deprived yourself of this experience, you still misunderstand something.

3. Cycling

Above, we discussed only the first cycle. If he did not give any result, then this does not mean at all that nothing will work out. Even if the techniques did not work, they still bring you closer to the phase state and you just need to try to do something further: turn back to the observation of images, phantom swinging and rotation. And so at least three more times. That is, after the first round of techniques, you can safely go to the second, third, fourth and even fifth. And all this during one waking up. It is very likely that on one of these cycles some technique will suddenly manifest itself, although it did not manifest itself a few seconds ago. Also, with new cycles, some changes in techniques are allowed. For example, you may feel that it would be better to replace seeing images with listening. Or you may feel that you are too alert, why you can alternate techniques with power sleep, etc. The main thing is to continue active actions and not lose chances, squeezing the maximum out of each situation.

Attention my friend! To avoid disappointment, you should set yourself the task of doing at least four cycles. The problem is that it is psychologically difficult for a person to do something that has shown itself to be inoperative, and he refuses to take further actions, although he could easily get into the phase. It must be remembered that from a quarter to a third of all indirect techniques work after the first cycle. There are even cases when a cycle from the second ten turned out to be effective, but you don't need to do anything for more than a minute. If it doesn't work, then it won't go, most likely, and further.

4. Falling asleep

All of the above referred to one awakening, that is, one attempt. If nothing happened during this time, it is much better to fall asleep again, so that when you wake up, make another attempt, and then another and another. This is how, for example, a whole series of successful experiences of the phase is accumulated in one morning. Moreover, it is very important to fall asleep with the clear intention of making an attempt a little later, since this greatly increases the likelihood that the next attempt will really be soon, and you will not just continue to sleep. That is, you do not need to fall asleep with an empty head and a desire to just sleep. If this concerns a deferred method, then a similar item is required, because there can be many attempts. The described four steps, if carried out accurately and consistently, will surely lead to getting into the phase in just a few attempts. If not, look for errors. Also, in order to use indirect cycles with greater efficiency, you need to know how to act if some technique suddenly started working, but after a while the dynamics stopped, and the phase did not come.

For example, you need to understand that if something has started to work, only a temporary lack of experience and skills will not allow you to reach the phase. Such barriers are overcome by temporary distraction to other techniques. For example, if the noise during listening increased and increased and suddenly stopped, it would be useful to be distracted for a few seconds, for example, by forceful falling asleep or observing images, and then return to listening again. At this point, the noise can get much louder and you can act accordingly. Sometimes it makes sense to interrupt several times for different techniques, but always return to the main one.

You can perform two or even three techniques at the same time. The result will not be affected. It is also normal and natural to switch from technique to technique outside of the action plan. For example, phantom wobble often generates noise. In this case, you can easily switch to listening.

I also want to warn you that at the first attempts you will encounter a memory problem. Having learned this whole algorithm, you can completely forget what exactly and how you need to do at the right time. Do not get lost. Do whatever comes to mind. In the process, you will remember your plan exactly. Moreover, even this chaotic action can give a result, because the main thing is not to waste time.

Brain Clues

As has been pointed out many times, my friend, variations in the cycles of indirect techniques are almost a must for maximum results. However, there are some exceptions. Sometimes, by indirect signs, you can understand that you need to start with certain techniques, regardless of what was originally planned. These are some kind of body tips. The ability to use them plays a very important role in indirect techniques, as it allows you to significantly increase the effectiveness of attempts and increase the total amount of practice.

Images

Waking up, you can immediately notice that you have some images before your eyes, pictures, the remnants of a dream. In this case, you need to start the technique of observing images with all the consequences that follow from it. If this does not lead to anything, then it is necessary to proceed to the cycles.

Noises

Also upon awakening , you may notice internal noise, hum, ringing, whistling, etc. Naturally, you need to immediately start with the listening technique. If in the end it does not give anything, it will be necessary to perform cycles of indirect techniques.

Vibrations

If, upon waking up, you feel vibrations in the body, then you need to start by strengthening them by tensing the brain or without muscular tension of the body. As soon as the vibrations reach a maximum, you can try to separate. If after several attempts nothing comes out, you should start performing cycles.

Numbness

It is also possible that you will wake up from time to time with numbness in different parts of the body, often without cause. As needed, immediately begin to do phantom rocking in the numb part of the body. If after some attempts this does not work, you can start quoting. Naturally, if the numbness is severe and causes significant discomfort, it is better not to use any techniques at all, but to take a comfortable position and then only try.

If the technicians finally wake up

In practice, you will notice that with unsuccessful attempts you encounter such a consequence as a transition to falling asleep or, conversely, to full bright wakefulness. As a rule, this indicates either a lack or an excess of activity, aggression. Your goal is to learn how to maneuver between these two extremes. It is between them that there is a phase. In practice, everything is very simple: if it is noticed that most attempts end in falling asleep, it means that more aggressive, accentuated and attentive actions are clearly lacking. This needs to be corrected right away. But the problem is much worse and more difficult if, on the contrary, most attempts end in complete awakening. In such cases, it is necessary to reduce activity and aggression, perform techniques more calmly, longer, as if falling asleep. Moreover, in each specific attempt, you should feel what exactly you need now more: passivity or activity. The relationship between these two extremes must be observed very clearly. Having begun your practice, you will return to this page more than once, since this is of essential importance and is often found in experience.

Even in successful practice, it happens imperceptibly that in reality success does not depend only on techniques. This is just one of the ingredients. After all, you can do them very carefully and actively, thereby only returning yourself to reality, which is useful when you initially want to sleep a lot or the body quickly turns off. But often it just wakes up. Understand that the phase occurs in your head, not in your body or because of some of your actions. If you only finally wake yourself up in reality with indirect techniques and do not approach the phase in any way, there is a very good option for changing the algorithm of actions. Waking up after sleep, before cycles of indirect techniques and before separation, trying not to move, immediately begin to do the power falling asleep technique for 3-10 seconds. You must very realistically and reliably for the body portray the desire to quickly fall asleep. How this is done - do not think. You have already applied it so many times in your life, and therefore intuitively you will do everything right. The signal will be a feeling of going inside yourself, almost falling asleep, but with the preservation of consciousness somewhere in the background of all this, so as not to fall asleep for real. Having made such a quick move, you will quickly and easily move your body to the phase state, which will make all further actions much more effective. The most interesting thing is that during awakening it may seem to you that nothing will work out and therefore you don't even have to try. Often, all efforts go more to combat such thoughts. You just need to do it, and often you will notice that, no matter how you evaluate the brightness of your awakening, just a few seconds of forceful falling asleep return you to a sleepy state. If you feel the effect well, then you can use such a forceful falling asleep simultaneously with all further actions, and not just before them.

Example from practice:

January, 2010 I woke up at about nine o'clock, and the first thought was that I woke up too brightly and nothing would work. As always, for some reason with difficulty, but I forced myself to try to do something - there was such a vivid feeling of awakening. The situation was aggravated by the physical movement - I was uncomfortable, and I rolled over on my stomach. I immediately fell asleep by force for a few seconds, which made me feel a sharp rollback of the state, as if I had gone a little deeper into myself. I immediately tried to separate, but nothing happened; no takeoff, no rolling out, no getting up. Started doing my favorite phantom swings. There was no movement. A few seconds later I tried hand visualization. Then observation of images. No result, although he noted that the hearing was muffled and I no longer clearly hear the sounds outside the window and around me. It definitely means something. I tried phantom rocking again, but after a few seconds nothing started happening. I decided to do hand visualization along with force falling asleep. He began to rotate his hands again in front of his forehead, rubbing his palms against each other, of course trying to see it all and at the same time seemed to fall asleep, leaving his consciousness into oblivion. Almost immediately I noticed that my hands were already less felt under the pillow, but more in front of my face. As soon as the consciousness was distracted by this, everything stopped immediately. He began to fall asleep again and try to feel and see hands in front of him. In the remaining awareness, I began to notice that the hands were more and more felt in front of the face and even began to appear. As soon as I realized that I could see them, I turned on all my consciousness and began to try to see them as clearly as possible. And in a couple of seconds they became visible in exactly the same way as in reality. At the same time, I completely felt them, even forgetting how and where they actually lie. By this time, no more than 30 seconds had passed since the moment of awakening. After that, I simply stood up, quickly making a plan of action in my mind. But suddenly the phone rang, which was lying on the floor near the bed. I took it in my hands, while feeling not only all its physical characteristics, but even the vibration of the melody. The number of a work colleague came up. I wondered what he would say to me in the phase, and I pressed the receive button. To my surprise, the phone still continued to ring. This caused confusion. I pressed accept again, but once again this did not lead to any result, and then I realized that the phone was ringing, it must have been in reality too. As soon as I thought about it, I instantly found myself in the body. The phone, however, rang, and indeed the same person called. It remains a mystery why this sound did not immediately knock me out of phase. Perhaps because of the logically ideal overlapping of spaces on top of each other.

Awareness in a dream

Dear friend, you should already know that the techniques for entering the phase through awareness in a dream are aimed at the emergence of awareness, complete self-understanding in the process of dreaming, which can lead to a full-fledged phase experience. Contrary to popular belief, techniques for entering the phase through sleep are not much different in nature from other techniques for entering the phase. The end result is still a dissociative experience in terms of its main indicators: it is full awareness and being outside the perceived physical body. The realism of the phase through awareness in a dream is also no different from that achieved with other techniques, and with deepening it can exceed the realism of everyday perception. This became obvious to the masses only in the 21st century, when the practice began to spread globally, and everyone can be convinced of the correctness of such a conclusion not on paper, but on experience. Always keep in mind in advance: if during a dream an understanding of the process suddenly arose, usually accompanied by a vivid thought "I'm dreaming!", then from that moment it is no longer a dream, but a phase.

But don't make the mistake that beginners usually make. Do not confuse the concept of awareness in a dream with the concept of controlled dreaming. Guided sleep is a sleep on demand, on a given topic, in which awareness is not implied. In addition, not everyone clearly understands what full awareness in a dream is. Many say that they are always aware of their dreams. That's bullshit. In part, awareness is always there, but you and I are talking about exactly the same consciousness as when we are awake. Not less. That is, in the presence of awareness, there can be no continuation of the plot of the dream. If there is a complete understanding that everything around is a dream, then the person abandons the plot and begins to do only what he wants right now. And after waking up, he should not think that the actions were absurd and inexplicable.

Naturally, when realizing in a dream, actions should not be chaotic, they should be completely subordinated to the desire to experience a qualitative phase. Therefore, having achieved awareness in a dream, one must immediately proceed to what would have to be done with both direct and indirect techniques, that is, deepening, retention, etc.

The actual techniques of awareness in a dream are very different in nature from any others associated with the phase, and it is not in vain that this direction often stands apart from the practices of the so-called astral projections and out-of-body travel, although all this is a phase. However, according to the final result, this technique hardly has any fundamental differences, as I have already noted. The peculiarities here are that in order to obtain a momentary result, it is not necessary to take specific actions. That is, all the technical elements are performed at a completely different time than the awareness itself. You probably understand this, because the reason is that it is impossible to perform any act if you are not aware of yourself and do not understand that you are dreaming. All efforts are spent on ensuring that this very awareness, for whatever reason, suddenly arises at least at some moment.

Due to the lack of direct effort, it is difficult to predict in front of the result when the lucid dream techniques will work. Although intensity and intent certainly have an impact on speed. Often, a realization in a dream can come literally at the very first fall into sleep, whenever it happens, or it can happen in two weeks or a month with everyday efforts. However, these techniques give greater guarantees of success than direct ones, and in terms of efficiency they can be compared with indirect techniques, yielding to the latter only in the speed of obtaining the effect and less effort. Moreover, if indirect techniques can be fully used only when there is an opportunity to sleep, then this does not play a significant role for awareness in a dream. Thus, to guarantee getting into the phase, you can safely use this technique, especially if there are any difficulties with other methods. But you need to keep in mind that there is much less direct control over actions than with any other techniques.

But in no case should you combine other types of techniques with awareness in a dream. It is better to focus on one thing at a particular time. Moreover, with the regular practice of any other technique, there is still an almost one hundred percent guarantee that awareness in a dream will occur spontaneously, and in any case, you need to know what to do if this happens.

Ways of awareness in a dream

Given the specifics of actions and the ultimate goal, several techniques can be used simultaneously to realize oneself in a dream. They are not only compatible, but can also complement each other. However, you can choose one and pay all your attention to it and get no less result. After all, the meaning is not in the number of actions, but in the amount of attention that you can give them.

Intention

The key, in fact the most important, is the increased inner desire to experience awareness in a dream. Intention itself is extremely important for any techniques related to the phase, but in this case it can be of the most basic importance. The creation of intention is connected with the creation of an internal desire, which manifests itself in both conscious and unconscious factors. Moreover, a strong intention is actually a kind of programming of the situation. The essence of the technique is in the formation of a strong desire to realize oneself in a dream. This desire should be developed both during wakefulness and immediately before falling asleep, which is even more important. Before a night, morning or afternoon sleep, you just need to really want to realize the dreams that are coming at all costs. It is advisable not only to want this, but also to think over what actions you will take in a successful case, how and for what it will be possible to use this situation. So you still need to be motivated.

remembering dreams

You must have come across the opinion that not every person has dreams. However, this is one of the most famous and common misconceptions. This simply cannot be. The problem is not at all that someone does not see dreams, but that not everyone remembers them. Even the one who sees dreams remembers only a small part of the dream upon awakening. That is, you should not think that if you do not remember dreams, you will not be able to realize yourself in a dream. You just have to try different techniques. Although, of course, this complicates the situation. There is a direct relationship between the likelihood of awareness in a dream and the number of remembered dreams. Therefore, the main technique, of course, is considered to be the development of the ability to remember dreams. In fact, everything rests on awareness, which is closely interconnected with the processes of memorization. In a dream, there is awareness, but it lacks fast, operational memory, so awareness of who you are, what your name is, how to walk, how to speak, will remain, but there is no idea how current events are related to those that happened a minute ago and what is their meaning. Think back to a couple of your last dreams and you'll understand what I'm talking about. However, by increasing the number of remembered dreams, we develop working memory in a dream, which allows us to first see more realistic dreams, and then, increasingly, lucid ones. And if so, then you can strive for this consciously. Technically, this is done in three main ways.

• Recall of all dreams upon awakening. Getting up in the morning, during the first minutes you need to remember as many dreams as possible that you had during the night. This must be done very carefully and diligently, since it is this technique that allows you to strengthen the crush. If possible, you need to remember these dreams in detail, or at least their main plots, already during the day or, even better, before a night's sleep.

• Recording dreams in a special diary is an even more effective way than simply memorizing and fixing dreams in your mind. This is also done in the morning, when the memories are still fresh. The more detailed the plot is described, the better it will affect the result. In addition, writing down greatly increases the awareness of actions and aspirations. The diary itself can be re-read from time to time to recall old dreams.

• Creating a kind of dream map (the so-called dream cartography) is an unusual way of remembering dreams. It is similar to keeping a diary, but here an increased level of awareness is achieved by trying to integrate all the plots when drawing up a map. First, one dream is recorded with a description of the scene of action, which is marked on the map. Then another one, and so on. When several dreams are recorded, a plot will necessarily be drawn up, which in one way or another will be connected with the place of the dream, which has already been described. These two close (according to the scene) dreams are marked on the map side by side. Over time, there are more and more such dreams, and the map becomes more and more complete. As a result, both the number of remembered dreams and their realism increase, and gradually awareness comes more and more often. It can also be assumed that the card is linked into one whole, not so much because it really exists, but so much because there is such a goal and this is inevitably reflected in the dream. It is even better to fix dreams in memory not at the final awakening, but at a temporary one. Waking up, the practitioner notes on a piece of paper with one phrase or even key words the plots of the last dreams, and then falls asleep. Then, by clues, most of the recorded dreams are recalled. The result of applying the technique of remembering dreams manifests itself first in the form of a rapid increase in the number of simple dreams themselves. When there are many of them, awareness begins to arise regularly.

Dream analysis

It helps a lot to be aware of oneself in a dream by constantly analyzing dreams in order to identify the cause of the lack of awareness, which is good to combine with recording dreams. The fact is that throughout a person's life, his consciousness gets used to the paradoxical nature of dreams, to which he does not pay any attention. This is expressed in the inability to understand, for example, that a red crocodile not only cannot speak, but cannot be red at all and be in an apartment. In a dream, we almost always treat such things without surprise. The essence of analysis is precisely to remember the dreams seen during the night and think carefully about why the paradoxical things were not adequately recognized. The daily analysis of dreams for their correspondence to reality every day begins to be reflected in thinking directly in a dream. For example, the same red crocodile immediately begins to cause doubt, prompting reflections that can lead to the understanding that everything around is a dream.

Creating an anchor

Awareness in a dream is not associated with specific actions in a dream, and habitual perception continues to work, so an artificially created conditioned reflex can be used. The technique consists in accustoming the mind to respond in the same way to certain stimuli that occur both during wakefulness and in a dream (necessarily both there and there). In other words, it is an attempt to create a habit of doing something in a certain situation. For example, in wakefulness, you need to ask yourself the question "Am I dreaming?" every time if an anchor appears in front of your eyes. This anchor can be any object that occurs relatively often both in wakefulness and in sleep: one's own hands, red objects, water, etc. At first, the practitioner is not always able to ask himself this question when he meets the agreed anchor. but through training and striving, he soon succeeds in doing it quite easily. Some more time passes, and out of habit, a person unconsciously begins to ask himself the same question when he meets the anchor not only in wakefulness, but also in a dream, which leads to awareness.

Of course, you must clearly understand that you need to not just ask yourself the question "Am I dreaming?" It is important to answer it carefully, trying to move away from the surrounding events so that the answer is as objective and unbiased as possible. Otherwise, even asking yourself this question in a dream, you will give the same answer as in wakefulness, that is, already incorrect ("I am not sleeping"). You can try to take off every time you answer a question. In reality, the attempt will be unsuccessful, but in a dream, most likely, it will succeed, which will once again prove that what is happening is a dream.

natural anchors

Fortunately, in addition to creating intentional anchors that, when trained, can induce dream lucidity, there are natural anchors. These are the objects and activities that most often cause awareness in a dream, even if there is no desire to achieve it. The very understanding of the existence of such anchors doubles the likelihood of their manifestation. Interestingly, this affects ordinary people many times less than practitioners. For the most part, these are such experiences in a dream as one's own death, acute pain, severe fear, stress, flight, electric shock, sexual sensations, vibrations, a dream about a phase and a dream about entering a phase. When training to deliberately achieve lucidity in a dream, these anchors should work almost 100% of the time.

Actions after waking up in a dream

Unfortunately, I have to repeat the same things so many times, but people still do not assimilate them, which is why I am forced to focus on this issue again. So, in order for awareness in a dream to lead to a full-fledged phase experience, it is necessary to know what options for action are available in this case. There are three main options:

• Immediately after awareness, proceed to deepening techniques, which should be done in any case first of all, as in the application of other techniques. Deepening is carried out right in the place of the plot. This will help to almost guaranteed to cling to the phase. Then you need to act in accordance with the plan of action in the phase. This is the best option, and I advise you to use it.

• Without a preliminary deepening, you can try to return to the body in order to immediately roll out of it in your room. There is a probable danger that, having easily returned to the body, one may no longer be separated from it, since the phase becomes much weaker if the physical sensations coincide with the position of the real body. If this option is nevertheless applied, then in order to return to the body, it is often enough just to think about it - and the movement occurs almost instantly. I strongly advise against doing this, but many people stubbornly try to do it this way, because they believe that in doing so, a lucid dream turns into an out-of-body experience. There is little sense in such reasoning, since it is easy to see that the properties of space and your possibilities do not change at all.

• When lucid dreaming, you can immediately apply moving techniques in order to get to any desired place. However, without initial deepening, it is also dangerous to use this option of action, since moving during a non-deepened phase is fraught with a return to wakefulness if the practitioner still has poor control over the intention, which by itself can hold. That is why the displacement is very often associated with an additional drop in the depth of the phase state.

Example from practice:

June, 2001 Just suddenly there was an awareness of being in a dream. I experienced feelings of joy and satisfaction. There were so many positive emotions that, realizing his position in the non-existent real world, he tried to share his emotions with a stranger. It didn't even matter to me that it didn't make sense. It should be noted that I did not have to return to the body in order to deepen the state and disconnect again, as I usually had to do, because there was immediately an atypical reality of everything around, because of which my awareness of being in a dream occurred.

I was in an extremely curious place: there was no sky - instead of it there was a large blue low dome, which spread a strange light evenly throughout the space; with its landscape, everything around resembled a kind of paradise, in which there were many fountains, streams and many architectural buildings of unknown purpose. Everywhere there were many manifestations of flora and fauna: all the streams were seething because of fish of different species teeming in the water, a lot of outlandish birds chirped and sang on all the trees (from simple green parrots to birds of fantastic appearance). As long as the view was enough, the most beautiful flowers and trees of the most bizarre forms were planted everywhere; there were a lot of people around, doing completely different things, not paying any attention to me; everywhere there were many different objects with known and unknown functions. Everything was distinguished by a great saturation of all possible manifestations of being. Everything was crowded, occupied, and there was almost not a single free place left. Everything literally boiled over. However, there was enough space to move around. I was overwhelmed with vivid emotions from such an unusual and, most importantly, realistic and clear landscape. Everything could be seen in the smallest detail. Due to the fact that there were a lot of things around, and I examined all this with interest, that is, I carried out concentration, I did not even have to think about the retention procedures. I didn't want to do what I had planned. I didn't need anything else, just to enjoy the simple observation of this piece of paradise. I felt like an alien in some strange world and was very happy that in life it happened that I could get into such a place. For this I was sincerely grateful to the phase. This would never happen in real life. Once again, from time to time it seemed to me that this was not my inner world at all, but some very real one, but the laws by which it flowed spoke of the impossibility of this. The only thing that could scare me in this situation was the reality of what was happening. My inner world can never get used to such things, because all my life I thought about everything in a completely different way.

The danger to my being in this paradise was the possibility of blackout and subsequent falling asleep. I began to worry a lot about it, so I had to do some more active things so that my consciousness would not drown. Without thinking twice, I decided to engage in communication with people, because this topic is always the most interesting there. Unfortunately, everyone who was present there was not familiar to me in reality. But this did not upset me much, because an interesting scene began to develop before my eyes. Two men began to sing songs, before that they sat quietly on the sidelines and drank an unknown liquid from a wineskin. From the tone of their voice and appearance, one could easily guess the alcoholic reason for their vocal concert. Having sung some excerpts from famous songs, they switched to obscene ditties and jokes. That's when the fun began. It was to be expected that they would only say things known to me, but, to my great surprise, this was not so. I stood and listened very carefully, although the ditties were funny, but I was not laughing - I had never heard them before . And this means that at this moment my brain is literally on the go creating quite high-quality things without my intervention in the process. Maybe everything that I heard in this world was once somewhere by chance in real life, but did not deserve my attention for any reason, and now in this form it was presented to my attention. Suddenly, the idea came to my mind that I need to have fun in a more active and unusual way, because I need to seize the moment ...

Direct technique

You should have already learned that direct techniques for entering the phase are carried out without prior sleep, by performing certain actions in a lying position with your eyes closed. Sleep is no longer needed here. At least in the way you are used to . The good side of this technique is that in theory it can be carried out at any time, and the big disadvantage is the duration of its development. Only every second can count on the appearance of an effect within 3-6 weeks with everyday attempts. For others, difficulties are not ruled out, to the point that no effect may occur even in a year. The problem is not that these techniques are not available to someone due to the natural characteristics of the body, but that not everyone can clearly understand certain technical nuances that we will talk about. It's always interesting to see that most tend to master these techniques in the first place, as they seem to be the most convenient, understandable and concrete. But a person who starts with this is 90% doomed to complete failure. Moreover, a lot of time will be lost, a lot of efforts and emotions will be spent. As a result, complete disappointment is possible in the entire sphere of phase experiences. To avoid such injustice, try not to make this mistake. It is worth starting the practice of direct techniques only after mastering the easiest indirect techniques or awareness in a dream. In any case, this will make it possible to reliably verify that the phase is not an invention. Moreover, the preliminary mastery of other techniques makes it easier to achieve direct entry into the phase. There are a number of other reasons why it is worth learning direct techniques only by having practice with other types of techniques. You just have to understand that this is aerobatics.

As already noted, direct techniques do not differ in the quality of experiences from indirect ones, which is also worth keeping in mind if you have just come to this. In addition, this phase is often of poor quality if the technique is performed late in the evening or at night, as the body requires a complete shutdown of consciousness and for this reason it is very easy to fall asleep. However, this is not true for everyone and not always. There are certain types of people who are more suited to direct techniques, but don't expect to be in that 10%. But indirect techniques are available to absolutely everyone and always.

Direct techniques do not always give quick and clear results. In the beginning, it may even be random. Therefore, it is impossible to start the practical path with direct techniques; one should not underestimate their complexity. You should not hope for a quick result in direct techniques. The main thing is to systematically work on technique, improving your skills from day to day. If even after a month of almost daily attempts no result has been obtained, you still need to keep trying and improving. Moreover, failures are always due to specific and understandable mistakes.

In no case should you abandon what was obtained before the use of indirect techniques, otherwise you can generally lose experience for a while - for example, the skills of their application themselves. However, you do not need to combine both on the same day. This will defocus attention and emotions. It is better to practice these two different types of techniques separately on days - for example, on weekdays, perform direct techniques before going to bed, and on weekends, catch moments of awakening for indirect techniques.

Time to Perform Direct Techniques

Of great importance is the time when direct techniques are performed. Although this also matters with indirect techniques, the main thing is that there should be an awakening. Here the conditions are much tougher. With direct techniques, the main difficulty lies in the initially too active state of consciousness, which is extremely difficult to turn in the opposite direction at any time you want. But there are a few time windows that will help you.

The best method for doing direct techniques is the delayed method. This is almost the same as with indirect techniques, but with some significant differences. Firstly, you can interrupt sleep at almost any time of the night and early morning. Secondly, after fixing the awakening, you do not need to fall asleep, but immediately proceed to the techniques. With the delayed method, direct techniques are several times more effective, because the brain does not yet have time to wake up 100%, a person easily falls into altered states of consciousness, and tangible results can be obtained on this wave. For example, you need to wake up in the middle of the night on your own or by an alarm clock, then do something for 3-10 minutes and then go to bed and do the techniques. If there is a possibility that you will wake up too abruptly, and then you will not even have a sleepy state, then the interval between awakening and direct technique should be shortened, allowing fewer actions at this time. Also, direct techniques for entering the phase should be done before falling asleep at night, that is, when you go to bed. At this time, the brain requires turning off the body and consciousness to restore the forces expended throughout the day. This process can be used, making certain adjustments to it. For a beginner, the least effective use of direct techniques during the day, given the normal biorhythms of the average person. However, if fatigue has time to accumulate, then this can be used, as the body will try to go to sleep. This is especially suitable for those who are used to sleeping during the day.

Attempt intensity

Given the important factor that the amount of emotions that a person can spend on any enterprise is of great importance, you need to know the measure, especially in such a delicate matter as the practice of the phase. It makes sense to make only one attempt to use the direct technique per day. If this happens more often, then the quality of each individual attempt will decrease significantly.

A lot of people try to take everything in a hurry, bringing the number of attempts to a dozen during the day. It is not surprising that this not only does not give any result, but also leads to the fact that after a few days the desire to do anything at all in connection with the practice of the phase disappears. This should not be in any case, even if the effect cannot be achieved within a week or a month. One must persistently, wisely, constantly analyzing the process, continue to practice the techniques, making the necessary corrections. But no more than once a day! This is the only way to do everything qualitatively and for a long period with the desire to acquire a new skill.

It is also almost hopeless to try to get into the phase with the help of a direct technique if, when you lie down in bed, you only think that you will not fall asleep until you enter the phase as well. Such rudeness in relations with the fine structure of the brain does not bring anything good - only rapid emotional exhaustion. If everything could be done with this. And then after all, then someone will say that the technologies described here do not work ...

Remember forever: the tightest time frame for performing direct techniques (before bedtime or in the middle of the night) is only 10-20 minutes. And no more! It didn't work - no big deal. Sleep well, life is not over yet, and there will be other attempts, more successful, if you draw the appropriate conclusions. If more time is given to this, then the sleepy state is interrupted, as the brain relaxes in the process of performing the techniques and no longer needs to be restored so much. The result is insomnia. Almost always and for almost everyone, after an hour of trying, sleep does not come for several more hours. This causes negative emotions not only because of the time spent falling asleep, but also because of unsuccessful attempts, a constant desire to sleep the next day, etc. As a result, a continuous negative is formed, and nothing else.

Position of the physical body

If you remember, buddy, in the case of indirect techniques, the initial position of the body did not matter, since the main thing was just to wake up, no matter how. But in the practice of direct techniques, this can be very significant. Separate failures arise due to the adoption of the wrong posture. I would even say that if a person does not know what is described below, then it was probably a major mistake in his previous attempts. The catch is that all people are different, and each person faces different situations every day. That is why there is no clear rule about what position of the body should be taken. There are certain recommendations that allow you to choose this very position, taking into account indirect signs.

Most firmly believe that you need to take a "dead man's position" (lying on your back, without a pillow, with legs and arms straightened). Perhaps this idea is borrowed from other practices of changing states of consciousness. However, it is this position of the body that harms most practitioners. This posture should only be taken if there is a chance that you will fall asleep quickly during the technique. In this case, this position should be uncomfortable for sleeping. If a person has problems with sleep and is always alert during the execution of direct techniques, he should take the most comfortable position, the one that seems most convenient at the moment. For some, paradoxically, it is the "corpse pose" that will turn out to be the best.

In general, remember the most important rule: the more likely you are to fall asleep, the less natural position of the body you need to take for sleep. The brighter the consciousness during the implementation of techniques and the worse the usual falling asleep, the more comfortable the position of the body should be taken. Depending on the situation, you can lie down in different ways and even be in a semi-sitting position. You may have to change your posture from attempt to attempt, making adjustments related to the floating state of consciousness, which will be discussed a little later.

Relaxation

Friend, you need to clearly understand that direct techniques themselves are relaxation techniques, because without relaxation there can be no phase. In addition, since the most effective time for using direct techniques is before bedtime and at night, and this is only 10-20 minutes, it is hardly worth spending extra time on relaxation or carving it out of these minutes. Moreover, correct and high-quality relaxation is a very delicate matter, but many people approach it casually and as a result get an effect completely opposite to relaxation. For example, they want to relax the body so much that the brain becomes so active, as if solving a complex mathematical equation. Is that the steam from the ears at this moment does not go. There can be no talk of any phase here. After all, the main thing is not the body at all. The body will always relax automatically when the mind is relaxed. And the body, in turn, will never relax if the brain is active.

And that's not all, instead of some kind of mechanical relaxation, I always like to just lie down for a couple of minutes, think about something, dream about something. This will be the best relaxation for the vast majority. The fact is that in this way the natural processes of relaxation are activated, and they are the strongest and deepest. For example, rarely does anyone relax to fall asleep, and sleep is also a highly altered state of consciousness. Without worrying about anything , relaxation can be applied only to those who know well what it is. As a rule, these are people with extensive experience of being in trance, meditative states. But in this case, relaxation should not take more than 1-3 minutes. There is no need for more, since anyone who knows how to relax knows that it is enough to think about relaxation just to think about how it comes. If you didn't remember this during practice, then this option is definitely not for you.

I would also like to note one more amazing thing: almost any high-quality relaxation techniques can serve as direct techniques in themselves, if a floating state of consciousness arises during their application. Therefore, with proper experience in working with them, you can also experiment in the direction of conquering the phase. Conversely, direct phase entry techniques can serve as excellent relaxation tools.

Options for using direct techniques

Do not get confused, for the direct entry into the phase, all the same techniques are used as for the indirect one, but according to a different principle of implementation. However, due to the fact that passive actions are more necessary when entering the phase directly, not all of these techniques are equally well suited. For example, such active techniques as brain tension are inapplicable for a smooth entry into the phase. True, they can shoot after leaving the "failure", but not about that yet.

If we talk about the process of performing direct techniques, then they differ from indirect ones in that the effect can be weak from the very beginning to the end of the attempt. But if, upon awakening, one of the techniques somehow showed itself, it can almost certainly lead to entering the phase, if you have not forgotten. That is, for example, phantom swinging with a direct technique can start quite quickly, but the amplitude will not progress, and the entire execution of the technique will be reduced to a rhythmic long movement. The effect of the appearance of the phase may appear not after 10 seconds, but after 10 minutes. The same goes for any other technique. Let me remind you once again that during indirect techniques you are already almost in the phase, if such a movement has arisen, at least a little. Significant difference, isn't it, my friend?

The main difference between direct and indirect techniques (directly in their implementation) is that they require different amounts of time. If with an indirect entry into the phase, as a rule, the testing time of any technique takes only 3-5 seconds, then in the case of a direct entry, it takes several minutes. And this time varies depending on certain factors. By the way, here you also have to choose 3-4 most suitable techniques, which I have described to you in the context of indirect methods of entering the phase. So, the main options for using direct techniques.

Classic variant (passive variant)

With one attempt - one technique. Techniques can be changed in different attempts. Applicable:
• at the initial stages;
• with difficulty falling asleep;
• if attempts lead to wakefulness;
• if attempts when using other options pass without failures of consciousness;
• if the body and consciousness are in a rested state.

Alternation (intermediate option)

With one attempt, two or three techniques for 1-5 minutes each. Techniques change little in different

attempts. Activity varies due to the duration of the techniques. Applicable:
• if, when using the classic version, falling asleep occurs, and when cycling - too bright wakefulness;
• during rapid normal falling asleep.

Cycling (active option)

The cycling of the three main techniques is the same as with an indirect entry into the phase, but not for 3-5 seconds, but for 10-60 seconds. Applicable:
• if the classic version and alternation lead to falling asleep;
• at the general extremely fast falling asleep;
• against the background of severe fatigue of a long lack of sleep.
Always practice direct techniques should begin with the classic version - one technique for the entire attempt. Due to the unusual nature of the actions, it may first happen that strong emotions force you to remain in a state of absolute wakefulness. But after a couple of days, sharp failures in sleep can begin without a quick return back. Therefore, it may be necessary to increase the dynamics by switching to interleaving.
Keep in mind that alternation is a prime use case for direct techniques, as it can be applied
differently. It itself can be passive if used for 15 minutes, alternating between two techniques of 5 minutes each. It can also be quite active if you alternate three techniques for 1 minute. Everything between these two extremes allows you to work correctly with techniques, choosing the best option for a floating state of consciousness.
Well, even if in the active form of the alternation there will invariably be a quick fall into sleep, you need to use

a cycle of indirect techniques, but with a wider time range - from 10 seconds to 1 minute, and not 3-5 seconds.

It is very important to understand that this involves a lot of work with techniques, and this can get tiring after a few days. Therefore, you should not torture yourself if you don't want to do something. Everything should be exclusively for pleasure and without excessive emotional stress. You should literally enjoy the very process of working with techniques. It should be very interesting, it really is. Outwardly, it may seem that this cannot be related to the effect. I wouldn't have believed it myself if anyone had told me about it a few years ago. But in practice, the direct dependence of the success of performing direct techniques on how pleasant it is to work with them is easily confirmed.

floating state of mind

Well, friend, now we come to the most important thing regarding this topic. To that, without which all the previous pages have no weight. As with indirect techniques, you must understand that the direct path to the phase consists of more than just techniques. Moreover, they are even more of secondary importance here, you can even do without them at all. There should be a clear understanding in your head that the work will take place with two main tools: the techniques themselves and a special state of consciousness. Without the second, all your attempts will be in vain. Many do not know this, and why they cannot gain experience. No one has noticed before, but if you analyze most of the descriptions of the direct entry into the phase state - in the literature, in the stories of practitioners, on the Internet, at seminars, you can extract a huge amount of various information. Sometimes one description is radically different from another. What just does not happen, and as soon as it does not work! But in most cases, one and the same feature is observed - these are short-term lapses of consciousness, superficial falling asleep, which is included in the concept of a floating state of consciousness. As a rule, all unusual pre-phase or phase sensations appear after it. This is exactly the key that opens the most complex direct technique. These lapses of consciousness can be literally seconds, or they can last several minutes or even more than an hour, and then it is already closer to the indirect technique. Sometimes they are a simple turning off of consciousness and falling into darkness, and sometimes they are going into a full-fledged dream. They can be single and rare, or they can occur several times a minute. The bottom line is that during them, the brain switches to a different mode of operation, which is just easy to use for the phase, if you manage to resist full falling asleep. You must clearly understand that it is very difficult for consciousness to switch to other modes of operation without sleep and it needs a kind of switch that our consciousness interferes with. That is why it is necessary to get rid of it for some moments.

Naturally, not every failure of consciousness gives a phase. The hole must be deep enough. Therefore, after each unsuccessful failure, you need to create the next, even deeper one. But the main problem with such actions is complete falling asleep on dips instead of temporary. It takes technology to deal with this. By and large, they perform more of an auxiliary function and therefore may vary . for many , it will be a bolt from the blue, but in the context of a direct entry into the phase of the technique, you can generally not use it if you learn to make lapses of consciousness due to only one intention, purely your own will. Performing techniques in their various variations, you just need to learn how to maneuver between full wakefulness and final falling asleep with the help of them. Also, this or that position of the body is suitable for such maneuvering, which we have separately discussed with you. Not the last way to resist falling asleep is a strong intention not to do so. It is expressed in the fact that during the execution of the direct technique, the practitioner constantly thinks about not falling asleep, even if he falls asleep. You also need to give yourself the installation that as soon as the consciousness falls into sleep, awakening will immediately occur.

If the opposite problem arises - the absence of failures as such, then the following technical tricks can help here: full concentration of attention on the action or, conversely, reflections and dreams parallel to the execution of the technique. I personally almost always think about something else during techniques, unless I feel that I really want to sleep.

One way or another, almost always there is a problem with the complete shutdown on dips rather than the complete absence of these dips. It is worth noting that if for a long time direct techniques do not even lead to light naps or single failures, then some significant mistake has been made in the techniques or in the timing for their implementation. You can regulate the number of dips by choosing the position of the body, the time of day, and the version of the technique. But don't worry too much about it. Usually, literally in the very first attempts, practitioners begin to understand how to fail and actively experiment, trying to simply fall deeper and deeper each time.

Now let's see how the entry into the phase occurs directly. Firstly, against the background of a failure, some technique may begin to work well, as a result of which you will immediately fall into the phase. Secondly, after a failure, unexpectedly brightly, the closeness of the phase may begin to appear - through noise, vibrations and other phenomena. At this point, you can immediately switch to appropriate techniques, such as listening and brain tension. Thirdly, against the background of the exit from the failure, it can be quite easy to simply split up or quickly, based on preliminary signs, find some working technique. By and large, you don't need to think about all this especially, since once you make a deep enough "dive", you will immediately feel the phase and can easily separate (if you are not afraid, of course).

However, if nothing happens for 10-30 seconds after exiting the failure, it is worth seeking it again, but in a deeper form. And after the next failure, analyze the situation again, trying to apply techniques or separate. And so all 10-15 minutes, separated by this type of technique. In fact, failures of consciousness are not always necessary, which is why they occur far from 100% of cases. But striving for them plays a huge role, even if they are not achieved. Dips are not necessarily bright, they can be very short-lived and superficial. Sometimes people don't even notice them. Also, they may not be at all, which is especially common with the delayed method of their execution (in the middle of the night).

Concluding this topic, I will say my favorite phrase, which I always use in class, to add more emotions to understanding the issue of indirect techniques. So, as long as your head is clear and in control during the execution of direct techniques, you will not succeed. It is your consciousness that is the stopper of your happiness. Do not be stingy with losing it in places in order to get a fantastic reward.

Case Study
January, 2009
When I went to bed, I was in the mood to try to get into the phase with a direct technique. After lying down for a while in thought, thereby calming down and relaxing a little, he began to concentrate his attention on the imagined rotation around its longitudinal axis. The first minute it was impossible to scroll more than half. But then the rotation became full and every minute it became easier and easier. It turned in one direction, then in the other. Periodically, dips into drowsiness and superficial sleep began to appear. Coming back from them, I didn't even try to attempt a separation, as I didn't feel any symptoms of the phase. At some point, consciousness fell into unconsciousness for a longer period of time than before (almost fell asleep completely), and when I woke up, the rotation was somehow "dim". I increased it, and it seemed to start some kind of motor in me: my whole body hummed with vibrations, although the rotation itself was still imagined, and not real in perception, as often happens. Also heard noise. It became clear that if I was out of phase, then I was close to it, and for the first time I tried to roll out. It worked out without a problem. Moreover, I did not fall to the floor, but hung a few centimeters from it, as it seemed to me. Wasting no time, he abruptly stood in the middle of the room. I didn't see it, but I clearly understood that I was in it. I quickly began feeling the floor, the closet, the bed linen, my torso, etc. In general, I immediately felt that the phase was deep, although there was no vision. I did everything more out

of habit and to guarantee a long and confident phase. Especially recently there was a failure in consciousness, and it was necessary to fully wake up before proceeding with actions, otherwise you can easily switch off. After 5-10 seconds of feeling, vision began to appear. As soon as it appeared, I stared at my hands, looking at all the lines on the palms and fingers. The phase has become not just real in perception - it has become hyper-realistic. At that moment, he quickly set goals: to obtain information about learning and to conduct an experiment with the connection of the observed body in phase with the physical body on the bed. I didn't immediately remember what I wanted to do next, but I decided that while I was doing these tasks, I would remember the rest. All the thinking about the plan of action did not take even two seconds, and then I closed my eyes and concentrated on the wise old man. There was a sudden flight, and I quickly enough, in just a few seconds, found myself in some kind of shack, as if I had fallen into it from the wall. The elder was sitting with his back to me, so I quickly walked around him and immediately asked how I could improve my teaching technique at the seminars. I expected that certain technical tricks and tricks would be offered to me once again. Instead, he unexpectedly said that it is worth working more actively on the emotional component, on motivation, since many simply do not make the necessary efforts, because they do not quite clearly understand what awaits them and how interesting it is. Although the techniques are worth adjusting, it does not make sense at the moment, since people are not always motivated to perform them to the fullest.

Having received what I needed and postponing its analysis for later, I took the opportunity and asked a question regarding personal relationships with close people. However, the answer made me droop, and I forgot for a couple of moments, which was enough for everything to become blurry. Realizing that the holding techniques directly in this place are useless, he simply tried to hold on to the phase, grabbing the sage by the beard. As a result, I ended up in the body, and the hand still held the beard, which I vigorously kneaded so that the flow of sensations was as strong as possible. He moved his hand with a beard, almost effortlessly stood up. Feeling the close space with his free hand and realizing that the condition is quite stable, he began to peer into the hand with a beard, brought it close to his eyes. Vision began to emerge, and in a couple of seconds I could clearly see the space and the hand itself. In it lay a dense patch of gray hair. This made me laugh, but I tried not to be distracted and managed to resist. Immediately he began to carry out research on the connection of the body visible on the bed in phase with the real one. Perhaps the space of the phase itself decided to help me, since this time my body really lay on the bed, and this happened less and less often, although at first it was so with almost every out-of-body experience. Looking at myself once again was not very pleasant, something inside was a little repulsive and caused mixed feelings. Perhaps because the person I saw did not quite correlate with the way I feel myself. I started touching his legs, stomach, head. It did not cause any thrust into the stencil. On the contrary, in spite of all prejudices, this process deepened me and kept me in the phase, because there was a sensorization of sensations. At some point, touching and examining the face, I thought too clearly that it was me, and for a moment everything blurred, and I even felt someone's hands on my face. But then he was able to return to what he was doing, and continued with the same clarity.

Everything became clear. Then it dawned on me that I never remembered what else I wanted to do. It was very disappointing, but I had to obey the very first desire in order to do at least something, and not suffer the rest of the phase because of my poor memory.

The other day I watched a documentary about deep sea creatures, and this is caused by a strong desire to be somewhere in the depths and see something like this with my own eyes. He removed his hands from the face of the body that remained on the bed, closed his eyes and concentrated on the depth. At first it was a simple flight, and then I began to feel the increased resistance of space, some kind of viscosity. And the tinnitus that appeared during the flight became muffled and squeezed. All this was a little distracting from the concentration on the goal. Focused even more. There was a cold and pain in the ears. The whole body began to compress. The movement stopped, and I realized that I was in the water and not breathing. Despite the understandable fear, he nevertheless opened his mouth, took water into his lungs and began to breathe, experiencing extremely unusual sensations from this alone. He began to peer into the darkness before his eyes, and gradually it began to dissipate a little. I knew that I shouldn't be able to see at this depth if the laws of physics were followed, but I still hoped for sight. If anything, I was already ready to create a powerful flashlight. Darkness has been replaced by greyness. I began to see a bright bottom. About fifty meters above him, you could still make out some kind of space, and above it was complete darkness. A very unusual picture against the background of even more unusual sensations of a crushed body. As soon as I began to look at something, I immediately moved forward, barely moving my limbs. It was very difficult to walk, but it allowed me to sensorize sensations and thereby hold on. A few seconds later I saw a bright spot in the grayness above the bottom, which was approaching me. A few more seconds - and I realized that this is some kind of fairly large creature. It quickly approached, and it became clear that it was an incredible squid. His body was already near me, and the tentacles were still stretching in the distance. There was a feeling that it was some kind of alien creature. The squid began to circle around me, stunned by what was happening and the realism that accompanied it all. Imperceptibly everything began to blur, and then I don't remember anything.

Chapter Three

Consciousness in a parallel world

Perhaps, dear friend, you will not be ready for this, but it is not enough to take the consciousness out of the body in order to cognize the Highest Yoga. This is just the first step. You will understand this at the very first experiences of phase experience, when it turns out to be very short, vague or completely uncontrollable. First you need to bring the state to a deep form. Then you need to always remember about the technologies of its retention. And you always need to be able to manage this space, because it has its own laws and rules. And to enter there with the ideas and views of everyday life is simply stupid and fraught with many problems. So, carefully study the following information, as they are just as necessary for you in your path of cultivation as the technologies for separating consciousness from the body themselves.

State stabilization

Deepening principle

Deepening is a technology for bringing the phase to full realism of perception and awareness. A phase is not some clear and fixed state in which you either are or you are not. This is an area of states characterized by a transition from the usual perception of the physical body to complete alienation from it; at the same time, consciousness and realistic perception are preserved, but they are carried out in a different space. During this transition, all sensations may initially be the most superficial - for example, vision may remain vague or completely absent. You need to know what to do with all this so that everything becomes hyper-realistic.

My friend, take into account in advance that a full-fledged experience of a phase is necessarily characterized by no less realism than the surrounding world. Moreover, in almost half of the cases, practitioners note that the real world even pales in comparison with the colorfulness and detail of the phase space. This is true, and you will check it for yourself. When you enter the phase, you must reach just such a state, and only after that you can proceed to any other actions. Moreover, the realism that needs to be achieved concerns not only vision, but also all other possible perceptions. Until deepening is carried out, there will not be a complete habitual perception of space. Consequently, there will be no point in being in the phase at all and somehow using it. For example, why try to find a person there if you can't even see his eyes or it will all be somehow vague? However, in a significant part of cases, deepening in the phase will not be required, since initially not only full realism, but also hyperrealism can take place. Naturally, in such situations, the deepening stage can be skipped and the planned actions can be started immediately. But still, it is better to do it a little, since it is not only about the clarity of perception, but also about consciousness.

Deepening is also important for the duration of retention in the phase. If you take action without bringing the phase to full realism of perception, its duration will almost always be several times less than possible. At the same time, the properties of the space of the phase also depend very strongly on its depth. For example, when everything is blurry and fuzzy, the stability of objects is very weak. There is also a clear dependence of the degree of realism of the phase on the degree of its awareness, therefore, for the clear work of consciousness, it is also very important to initially go deep into the phase to the maximum. In general, there are many other reasons why the lack of deepening is always considered a gross mistake. It's funny, for a long time almost no one spoke or wrote about this most important rule, although you yourself will understand in practice that it is paramount. One can only guess how it happened.

Direct deepening should begin only after the final separation from the body. If it is started earlier, the phase may end. If for some reason the final separation from the body does not occur, it is necessary to achieve it at all costs in the first place. As for the deepening techniques themselves, there is one main technique and several secondary ones.

Sensory sensations

The basic rule of deepening in the phase and its retention is as follows: the more and longer you feel the phase with your senses, the deeper and longer it will be. Sensitization of sensations is the most effective deepening technique precisely because it allows you to activate the main sensations, thereby transferring a person from reality to a phase. After all, a person is, first of all, his feelings. There are several types of sensory perception.

Feeling

Vision may not be there initially, but the feeling of being somewhere is almost always there. Therefore, in such cases, you can be guaranteed to use only one type of perception - tactile-kinesthetic. That is, you can move and touch something at the same time. As you know, these sensations play a huge role in our perception of the world around us. Accordingly, if you actively invoke them with the help of the space of the phase, they will not only take you there, but they themselves will reach the maximum. The feeling itself consists in the fact that you need to immediately start touching everything around quickly. You need to do this quickly, but carefully, perceiving the felt surfaces and shapes. You can not keep your hands in one place for more than 1 second. They must feel something all the time, somehow move. In this case, it is useful not only to quickly touch objects, but also to briefly examine them by touch. If we talk about specific objects, then, having rolled out of the body, you can feel the bed, floor, carpet, nearby walls, table, etc. You can also use an interesting experience with rubbing your palms against each other, as if we want to warm them. At the same time, you can also blow on the palm of your hand to "turn on" additional sensations. It is also useful to quickly feel your sensed body in the phase. As soon as you start feeling, you immediately get the feeling that a deepening and fixation of the state is taking place. Usually it takes just a few seconds to achieve the maximum result. At this time, pseudo-physical sensations will be no different from everyday ones. If initially there was no vision, then, as a rule, during palpation it quickly arises.

Looking after

This technique is the most important technical type of sensorization of sensations. However, initially it is not always possible to apply it, since there may not be vision. If vision has appeared or has been created by special techniques, then you can start looking. The effect of this technique is due to the fact that vision is the main source of perception. Therefore, by irritating him with phase sensations to the maximum, you can completely disconnect from the real world. Do not forget that the more sensations there are in a phase, the more fixed it is.

Sighting should be done only from a distance of 10-15 cm from objects. At the same time, you need to try to quickly look at the small details of the objects that are around. For example, looking at the hands, look at the lines on them. Looking at the wall, pay attention to the texture of the wallpaper. Looking at the mug, peer into small details, inscriptions. You can not hold your attention in one place for more than half a second. The gaze must constantly sort out new and new objects and their details. It is quite normal not only to approach objects to examine them, but also to bring them to the eyes, if possible. It is desirable that the objects are not in different parts of space, but are nearby, otherwise you will have to spend time moving from object to object. As a rule, if the visibility was initially vague and a pull into the physical body was felt, then in just 3-10 seconds there is no trace of this. The effect of the technique is very fast and noticeable. The most important point in understanding this technique should be considered the desire to peer into small details from a close distance. That is, not just to look at them, but to peer: if you see - you peer into the next object.

Looking and feeling

This type of sensorization affects the most important instruments of human perception, so the effect is at least doubled compared to the effect when performing each of these techniques separately. In fact, this type of technique should be started without fail if there is vision in the phase. This will allow you to get a good phase depth faster and with less force. It is best to perform palpation and looking not only simultaneously, but also in relation to the same objects (for example, looking at hands, simultaneously rubbing them against each other). You also need to observe the dynamics and do not forget that you need to get sensations not for show, but as sharply as possible.

Secondary Deepening Techniques

Falling upside down

This technique is used when the practitioner in the halyard is hovering in an undefined space where there is nothing to touch or look at. Its essence lies in unusual vestibular sensations that are abruptly disconnected from real physical perception. In the phase, you need to close your eyes, if, of course, you have vision, and literally dive head first into the floor or space below. When flying down, there will immediately be a feeling of moving away from the physical body, and the fall itself will be perceived as if it were happening for real. In parallel, darkening of space and cooling may occur. Anxiety or fear may also appear. After 5-15 seconds of such a flight, the practitioner will either be thrown to some indefinite place in the phase, or something like a dead end, a wall will appear in front of him. Then you need to apply the technique of movement. Also, movement can be used if during the flight there is no depression, or it has stopped progressing, or, according to sensations, has already reached the desired degree. In these cases, instead of using the movement technique, you can also simply bring your hands to your eyes at a distance of 10-15 cm and, without opening your eyes, try to see them. This will also lead to hitting some random place if there is no specific target. When falling upside down, you should not think about hitting the floor if there is a need to fly through it. You need inner confidence that the barrier will be overcome. In addition, if the phase is still shallow, such tricks are easier than usual.

Keep in mind that the mood is of great importance not just to fall down and observe the sensations, but to want to rush down sharply, trying to move away from the body. If this is not done, such a fall, instead of deepening, can lead to a return to wakefulness, that is, you have to start all over again. And this happens for the simple reason that if you fall down uncontrollably, relaxation may occur, and this always returns you to reality.

Representation of reality

This technique should be applied if there is a certain experience of entering the phase or if other techniques do not work. The point is to imagine, already in a state separated from the body and having vision, that you are not in a phase, but in the physical world with its inherent realism. You need to do this very carefully and aggressively, trying to literally feel your idea of everyday life. At this moment, the surrounding space will immediately begin to become brighter, and in just a few seconds, the realism of perception can reach not only the level of perception of the physical world, but even surpass it. If after a few seconds of applying the technique there is no result, it should be changed to another. However, if this happened, then the point is not at all in the technique, but in the fact that it was incorrectly applied.

Activity

It must always be remembered that when performing any deepening technique, activity is key. If everything is done calmly, imposingly and slowly, then instead of deepening, falling asleep or returning back to the body will more often occur. Any deepening technique must be performed very actively. The whole process should be somewhat hectic and aggressive. No stops, but only continuous attentive and active action.

Retention principle

Holding techniques help to stay in the phase for as long as possible. If you do not know these techniques, the duration of being in this state will be many times less than when using them. In the worst case, the phase may only last a few seconds. Usually beginner practitioners are concerned about the question of how to return from the phase, how not to stay there for a long time. However, in reality, such a problem does not arise at all, everything happens quite the opposite, and, perhaps, because for an organism, a phase is not a completely natural state. Retention is the main problem. You will understand this at the very first experiences of the phase.
The retention technique is divided into three main areas: counteracting the return to wakefulness (foul), falling asleep and false exit from the phase. As a rule, at the beginning of the journey, the first two problems are equally faced, but then the third begins to manifest itself. Although I increasingly meet people who are

tormented by false exits from the phase from the very beginning. For beginners, the resistance to returning to the body is usually immediately clear, but what is the opposition to falling asleep, many do not know. However, almost half of the phase experiences usually end in a banal falling asleep. It looks like this: a person loses attention, his awareness of himself in a dream disappears, and everything around gradually loses clarity, turns into an ordinary dream in all respects.

But if we talk about counteracting the false termination of the phase, then the situation here is much more surprising and dramatic. In some cases, the practitioner feels an impending exit from the phase (foul), but no holding techniques help, and he ends up in the body. At the same time, he clearly feels that there was just a phase, and now it is a familiar reality. Then he gets up and literally after a few steps falls asleep, because he got up not in reality. However, most often in such cases, falling asleep occurs without any movement, but right in bed. The problem is how vividly the difference between the phase and reality can be modeled, since it is almost impossible to distinguish the phase from reality by external and internal indicators. You need to know the mandatory actions in case the phase ends, since this can be a deception or a delusion, no matter how you really perceive it.

Of course, in some cases, retention techniques are not relevant. But at its core, knowledge of retention techniques is important for the vast majority of practitioners, no less than 90% of practitioners. It may also be that someone is faced with the need to counteract only a foul, and someone - only falling asleep. All this is very individual and is determined only in practice. However, you yourself will soon understand this. Usually you should count on 2-4 minutes of staying in the phase, even if you know all the techniques of holding to perfection. But do not think that this time is not enough. The peculiarity of the space of the phase is that achieving something and moving there takes a minimum of time, seconds, while in reality this is what most of the life is spent on. Therefore, in the same 3 minutes in the phase, you can do so much that you even need a list so as not to waste this time in vain.

It is also necessary to take into account the factor of personal perception of time and events. As a rule, a practitioner, especially a beginner, perceives one minute in a phase as 5-10 minutes of real time. This is influenced by the psychological characteristics of the personality, the unusual state of the brain, certain experiences and events in the phase. That is, it may seem to you that you were there for half an hour, but in reality it can take no more than a couple of minutes. To understand how long the phase actually lasted, you don't need to try to track the time in reality. It is better to calculate how many actions were performed in it and how long each of them could take.

The maximum duration of stay in the phase varies depending on individual characteristics, the ability to apply retention techniques and, possibly, the time of day. It is difficult for someone to reach the time barrier of 2 minutes, for someone it is easy to be in the phase of 10 minutes or more. However, the organism, as a rule, does not allow maintaining the phase for a long time - it is unlikely that anyone will be able to stay in the phase for even some real 20 minutes. True, according to personal subjective perception, they can stretch for many hours.

Foul Countering

Permanent sensorization

Exactly the same sensorization of sensations that was described in the context of deepening applies to retention. The bottom line is that, having reached the desired depth of the phase, do not stop irritating perception, but continue to do it all the time, albeit not in such an active form as when deepening. Throughout the entire phase, all your actions must be combined with obtaining the maximum amount of tactile-kinesthetic and visual sensations. That is, you should touch everything around and examine it in small details all the time. For example, when passing by a bookcase, you need to quickly touch and examine the books in it, details and corners. This is how you should behave at all times. Feeling can be used separately, as a background, that is, visual perception is freed from additional load, and hands constantly touch something, or even better, rub them against each other.

Sensory on demand

Sensing on the need for action is no different from constant sensoring, but is used only in those cases when a foul begins to be felt, that is, a return to wakefulness, or when everything around just starts to blur and lose clarity. In essence, this technique of holding is the application of a regular deepening, if necessary, when you begin to feel a sharp drawdown in the clarity of space, which usually happens before a foul. At this moment, you need to abruptly begin to feel everything around, examine it in detail, etc. As soon as the environment becomes clear and realistic again, you can continue actions without sensorization.

Constant vibrations

Now we are talking about the constant maintenance of strong vibrations in the phase. Vibrations directly in the phase are almost always easily achieved by simple tension of the brain or non-muscular tension of the body. Having created them in this way, you can continue to hold them, which will have a positive effect on the time spent in the phase. A fairly simple technique, given the important fact that your hands and eyes remain free.

Vibrations as needed

However, there is another option: vibrations are created and intensified only at the moment when there are signs of the termination of the phase; perception becomes ambivalent, sensations blurred. Strengthening the vibrations at this moment will allow you to go deep into the phase again, after which you can continue actions without them. With luck, this does not take more than a few seconds.

Force falling asleep

As soon as the signs of a foul appear, one should immediately lie down on the floor and try to force sleep, as in the phase entry techniques, but in the most direct sense. That is, you must literally lie on the ground or on the floor, wherever you are, and pretend to fall asleep. After lying like this for a few seconds, you can get up and continue your journey in the phase, since realism and depth will most likely be restored. The main thing is not to fall asleep for real.

Rotation

In contrast to the similarly named technique of entering the phase, in this case there is no need to imagine anything. You really need to rotate around your own axis in phase according to your perception. After a few turns, the depth will be restored, and you can continue to work. If signs of a foul remain, take a few more turns.

Check

Being in the phase, one should constantly try to count, striving to reach the highest possible value. It should not be a simple aimless counting in the mind - you need to strive for the maximum, count as long as possible. The score itself can be kept both mentally and aloud. This technique turns out to be effective due to a clearly expressed desire to stay in the phase longer due to the desire to count to the maximum possible value. A clear goal that has arisen helps even unconsciously to perform the actions necessary for a long retention in the phase.

Phase lock

Undoubtedly, one of the most interesting ways to stay in the phase is the ability to cling to it. This must be taken in the most literal sense. At the moment of an approaching foul, in the phase, grab something with your hands and actively feel this object or squeeze it. Even when the return to the body takes place, the hands held the object from the phase, and will continue to hold it, but the real hands will not be felt. Starting with these phantom hand sensations, you can separate again or create a full phase. You can grab any objects that are nearby: a chair leg, a glass, a doorknob, a stone, a stick, etc. If there is nothing around, it is better to simply clasp your hands, bite your lip or tongue. Most importantly, it should not be a passive action. If you already clasped your hands, for example, then wrinkle them together, three, etc. Do not forget - it is always a matter of sensations, their number.

Sleep resistance
Constant awareness of the likelihood of falling asleep

Remember, most of the falling asleep in the phase can be overcome with the help of a simple understanding that such a development of the situation is very possible. The practitioner in the phase should always keep in the background the thought of the probability of falling asleep and therefore carefully analyze each of his actions: to what extent it is carried out due to real desires, and not paradoxical ones, as happens in an ordinary dream or on the eve of it.

Periodic Mindfulness Analysis

In the most severe cases, you need to periodically ask yourself the question: "Am I sleeping?" Mentally answering it, you need to carefully assess the situation and the adequacy of the current actions. If everything corresponds to the norms of awareness, actions continue. If the practitioner sets himself the goal of asking this question regularly, sooner or later the question will pop up by inertia at the moment when consciousness really falls into sleep. Then this will help the consciousness to wake up, after which it will be possible to continue to be in a full-fledged conscious phase.

The interval that should be between questions should be chosen based on the individual's ability to stay in the phase. If the phase usually lasts a long time (5-10 minutes or more), you should not try to ask a question more often than once every 2 minutes. In other cases, it makes sense to ask a question often, literally once a minute or even more often.

Anti-Unrecognized Phase

Because phase completion reality testing techniques can be somewhat silly and require extra attention to the actions being performed, they should only be used when necessary. Until then, they need only be kept in mind and used only in moments of doubt. Using the same methods, you can definitely determine whether you are in the phase with techniques for entering it.

Hyperconcentration

As already noted, the cessation of a phase experience can be simulated and in no way differ in perception from the state when the phase actually ends and the practitioner returns to reality. Therefore, it is necessary to look for a way out, based on the differences between the spaces of the physical world and the phase. That is, you need to know how to unequivocally understand whether you are in the phase or not. There is only one practical method available that can always guarantee an accurate result; this way - hyperconcentration. The phase space cannot sustain a long period of close visual attention to the small details of objects. After a few seconds, they begin to distort, change color, smoke, melt, etc.

Upon exiting the phase, you need to look at a small object, some point, from a distance of 10-15 cm and keep your eyes on it for the next 10 seconds. If the object does not change, then reality is around, if it is somehow distorted, it is a phase. The easiest way is to look at the tip of your finger, some point on it or a scratch.

Minor Techniques

However, there are a number of methods for testing a foul for reality. Due to the fact that any situation, any properties and functions can be modeled in the phase, these techniques are not always applicable. For example, it is believed that it is enough just to try to do something impossible in reality - and if there is a phase around, it will manifest itself. In fact, the laws of the physical world can be modeled, and the same take-off, passage through the wall and telekinesis will not work even in the deepest phase. It is also suggested to look at the clock twice in a row - in the phase they will supposedly show different times. But this will not always be the case either.

Modeling can be 100% related to the everyday world around the practitioner, but in an expanded form it happens very rarely, so it is usually possible to understand whether you are in the phase or not by carefully examining the room in which everything is happening. As a rule, there will be something superfluous in it, something will be missing, the time of day or even the season will not match, etc. For example, with a false foul, there may not be a table with a TV in the room, or it will be, but in a different color. This should immediately serve as a signal.

There is one action that can often help to recognize the phase - exhaling through a pinched nose. In general, even in the phase you may not exhale through a pinched nose (if you are very sure that you are in reality), but often this helps. That is, in the phase, you can breathe even through a pinched nose, and the possibility of this will indicate the true state of things, if in doubt.

Moreover, there is an interesting logical feature. Despite the amazing similarity of the space of the phase and reality, if you still have thoughts that the phase continues, then, most likely, this is really a phase. Of course, this only applies to situations when you return from a phase and cannot understand whether it has ended or not. That is, it has little to do with entering the phase, when the beginner still cannot understand whether he is close or not. In this case, it's just the opposite. Such thoughts can be a sign that you are not close at all, especially when it comes to direct techniques.

Retention rules

Don't look into the distance

Remember, if you look at distant objects for a long time, a foul or movement to these objects can happen. To look at distant objects without problems, you need to simultaneously observe the elements of the holding technique - for example, periodically look at your hands in front of you, rub them against one another, maintain strong vibrations, etc.

Constant activity

A very important point: in no case should you be passive and calm in the phase. The more actions, the longer the phase. The fewer actions, the shorter the phase. It is worth stopping in thought - as everything stops right there.

Action plan

You need to have a clear action plan, consisting of at least four to five points. It must be consistently carried out in the phase during its closest experience. This is necessary for several important reasons. Firstly, in this case, you will not stop in the phase wondering what to do. Secondly, in order to complete all the assigned tasks, you will even inadvertently perform the necessary retention actions. Thirdly, meaningful and pre-conceived actions will allow you to always move forward, and not pointlessly waste phase experiences on what comes to mind at the current moment. Fourthly, the action plan creates the necessary motivation, therefore, additional intention for the implementation of phase entry techniques, which is often the determining factor. In other words, the action plan itself will even contribute to the frequency of entering the phase.

Inner silence

Less internal dialogue and thinking in the phase - you experience it longer. Thinking should concern only what is being carried out and felt, and talking with oneself is generally prohibited. The reason is that many thoughts in the phase can serve as a program, and even their inner pronunciation can make adjustments to the process, including negative ones. For example, thoughts about the body return to it. Also thoughts about the foul are returned to the body. A person can think and relax because of this, which will also lead to a foul. In addition, random thoughts usually easily lead to ordinary falling asleep.

Try to get out again

The most important rule: you should always remember that a typical phase experience does not consist of one entry into it and exit, but of several repetitions of such actions. In most cases, you can get into the phase again as soon as it has ended, if you try to apply the techniques of separation or creating a phase state immediately upon returning to the body. If the practitioner has just been in the phase, his state is close to it anyway, and you just need to apply the techniques to continue the journey. This can be tried again and again, many times within the same attempt. Only thanks to this point you can get several times more practical experience. Accordingly, without it, you will not advance as much as you could.

Case Study

April, 2002
After another awakening, I decided to try to get into the phase. There were no signs of a close phase, but it immediately turned out to roll out. Surprised by such an easy exit, he began to go deeper by feeling: first he completely searched the bed, and then the objects closest to it. Gradually, the sensations became more and more real. But the sight did not appear. Then I decided to go by feel, hoping that the vision would appear by

itself, as it always happened before in such cases. While moving around the apartment, after a few meters, fuzzy vision began to appear, which I easily deepened by concentrating on my hands. Instead of doing some productive activity, doing research, I decided to have fun. To begin with, it flew up sharply through several apartments at once, while experiencing an unforgettable sensation, flying through concrete floors. Then he repeated this movement in the opposite direction, but already to the first floor. During the flight through other people's apartments it was possible to look at the situation. There was a great temptation to engage in destruction in the apartment on the first floor, but even more I wanted to fly, and I flew headlong at an angle upwards through the wall into the street. He flew up about fifty meters and hovered in the middle of the yard. To maintain the phase, from time to time he looked at his hands, and only then examined the details of the landscape. The spirit was captured from the height. Birds flew by and the wind blew. I experienced a real thrill. At one moment I forgot a little, and almost lost the phase, but managed to create vibrations by exerting the brain. Subsequently, with the help of control over them, he was able to hold the phase for a long time without resorting to concentration.

Then a great idea came to my mind: I decided to try myself as a military fighter. Not without difficulty, he was able to concentrate on this goal and, sharply picking up speed, rushed to the side. The more the speed became, the more the hum in my ears became. With every cell I felt a frantic movement, crazy speed. Of course, it was possible to fly and feel only movement, but I deliberately tuned in to feel all the aerodynamic effects. The air with a whistle and growing warmth let me through it. I struggled to overcome my fear, which was left from the ordinary world. Clouds flashed above me, and below - houses, forests, people, and everything was so real that I really thought about what was happening, how to relate to it and what it is …

Space Management

As you understand, my friend, space cannot be used for any purpose without being able to move around and find the right things. If in wakefulness we know approximately where something can be and how to find it, then in the phase we cannot follow the same path, since all these mechanisms work there according to a different principle. In the phase, everything is much simplified . We consider moving in the phase and finding objects in it in one chapter, because these techniques are based on the same mechanisms. Almost all of them, with minor changes, can be used for both one and the other. Having studied these techniques, you can go anywhere and find anything in the phase. Such a breadth of possibilities must be understood only literally. The only restrictions in this situation are the breadth of fantasy and the strength of desires, as usual in a phase.

Of course, in connection with the movement, one should not focus on the ways of traveling in close spaces. For example, you can simply walk into the next room, and you can get outside along the corridor or through the window. All this is understandable and so. One should also focus on moving to distant spaces that are beyond the scope of rapid physical achievement. Keep in mind in advance that if the movement techniques fail, and you end up in the wrong places, you should immediately apply them again until the desired result is achieved.

One way or another, at first you will have to practice, so that later everything turns out easily. In the end, this is not a fantasy, controlled by one excitement of consciousness.

When it comes to finding objects, then objects are understood to be any particulars of space, both its inanimate and animate components. That is, these techniques are equally effective for finding both a person and an object. However, there are several techniques that are only suitable for finding living objects.

Movement Techniques

Teleportation with closed eyes

This is a basic movement technique that should be mastered in any case. Not to say that it is the simplest, but when it is mastered, very important skills for practice are worked out, which will come in handy many times. To use it, you need to close your eyes if you have vision, and then do just one thing - concentrate on the thought form, the image of the place you want to get to. Immediately there will be a feeling of a rapid flight, and after a few seconds there will be an ejection into the desired space.

The main difficulty lies in the ability to concentrate on one single goal - the desired place. This must be done very clearly, confidently, aggressively and without distraction. Any outside thoughts have an extremely negative effect on the performance of the technique. Because of them, the flight can be very long, end in a foul or ejection to another place. So you have to work hard during training.

Closed eye technique

This is one of the easiest techniques. You just need to just close your eyes, concentrating on a very bright thought that you will open them already in the required space. At the moment of closing the eyes, it is useful to imagine yourself already in the right place, which will greatly increase the effectiveness of the technique. The movement must take place here and now, and necessarily without flight, as in teleportation with closed eyes. You need to open your eyes at the moment when you are completely sure that you are already in the right place. And it can only take a second if you can practice. Remember, there is only one barrier here - your confidence.

Focus on a distant object

For this technique, you need to peer from afar into the small detail of the place where you would like to be. The more closely you try to see this detail, the faster the unexpected feeling will appear that you are already next to it. Of course, the only drawback of this technique is that moving is possible only to those places that are initially visible, at least from afar.

Moving while splitting

I think this is one of the best ways to travel. This technique is very simple and convenient to perform, and it can be used with almost any separation technique. The bottom line is that in the initial stages of leaving the body, you need to focus on the image and feeling of the place you would like to go to. It would be even better to imagine that you are already in it. As a rule, having divided, the practitioner ends up where he wanted to be. A huge plus of the technique is a significant time saving, because you don't have to think about moving to the first place where you wanted to go in the phase. However, a significant drawback of the technique is that the separation occurs only at the beginning of the experience of the phase, and therefore it will be possible to apply it only once. Then you should resort to other options.

Door technology

This is the most popular and simple technique. In the phase, you need to go to any door and focus on the fact that it leads to the right place. When you open the door, you will see this place in front of you and go into it. If the door was originally open, it must first be closed. But do not think that a simple desire is enough. Confidence that the right place behind the door should be exactly the same as when you come to the door of your apartment, knowing that your apartment is there. It can be problematic at first, but with a little practice it will be a lot of fun. It turns out that the door from your room where you sleep leads to all worlds in all universes. If you have experience, then you know that I am not joking. And if not yet, then, believe me, you will still be surprised in this life.
The disadvantage of the technique is that for its implementation it is necessary to have a door. If there is no door, lovers of this movement technique create it using the technique of finding objects or try another movement option.

Object Finding Techniques

Buddy, all moving techniques are also relevant for finding an object, since in both cases we are talking about changing space. But when finding objects with the same techniques and moving, instead of some place, you need to concentrate the will on a specific detail of the space that needs to be found. As a result, you will find the desired object, but it is not necessarily guaranteed to preserve the original place from where the action was performed.

But if your goal is to find an object, always being in the same place, you should use the specialized techniques described below, which allow you to change only a part of the space.

Finding a person by calling him by name

This technique is used only to find living objects. In the phase, you need to call the name of the person or animal you are looking for, expecting that this object will enter the room or somehow imperceptibly appear in it. You need to call loudly, almost shouting. As a rule, to achieve the result, it is enough to pronounce the name a few times. It doesn't have to be just sound. Put your desire into it, otherwise nothing will work. If the desired animate object does not have a name or its name is unknown, you need to shout out any name or simply repeat: "Come! Come!" The main thing at the same time is to focus on the image of the one you need to see.

Finding with a survey

For this technique, you need to approach any person in the phase and ask him how you can quickly find the desired an object. As a rule, the object immediately gives the right advice, after which you need to follow the instructions. It is important not to forget to ask how quickly this can be done, or to clarify in the question that the object is nearby, otherwise you can spend a lot of time. The fact is that you can be shown a too long way or some kind of time frame, like "come back in an hour." Also, in no case, when communicating with a person, you should not doubt his words, since this is fraught with the fact that he will lie, and you will not find anything or anyone. The disadvantage of this technique is the need for the presence of a person nearby and the ability to communicate with such objects in the phase.

Turning technique

To use this technique, you need to focus on the fact that the object you are looking for is somewhere behind you. Turning around, you will actually find an object there, although it was not there just a moment ago. Again, don't think it's as simple as these two sentences. You need to gain complete confidence that the object is really behind you, complete and all-consuming confidence. Any slightest doubt will spoil the result.

Finding around the corner

Always keep in mind that, approaching any corner in phase, you can concentrate and imagine that behind it is the desired object, animate or not. And turning the corner, you will see what you want. It is clear that any space visibility limiter can act as a corner. It is not only the corner of the house, but also the corner of the cabinet, the corner of the truck bed, etc.

The disadvantage of the technique is the need to have some corner of sufficient size, but this is not a problem, because you will still be in the phase most of the time in urban-type spaces.

Being in hand

This technique is only suitable for objects that can fit in the hand or that can be held by it. To implement it, you need to focus on the perceived feeling that the object is already in your hand. At this moment, you can not look at the hand. Soon after a clear concentration, there will first be a slight, and then a full-fledged feeling that the object is already in the hand. The technique should be carried out in such a way that the object is already in the hand, but for some reason you do not feel it. And it is during the attempt to still feel it that he appears.

Case Study January, 2004

The body was very tired, even though I managed to sleep for several hours at night. As soon as I lay down, I almost immediately felt the emerging vibrations, but I didn't have enough relaxation to turn them on with all my might. At the moment, the most convenient way to relax and enter the phase seems to me to be excitations (a floating state of consciousness). I turned out to be right, because already after the fifth or sixth time I sharply felt vibrations grabbing me from all sides. In this case, there was no need to strengthen or deepen them, since the body is tired, and it will create the deepest possible state on its own in order to quickly restore vitality. I just lay there and watched the changes taking place with me, but you can't stay inactive for a long time so as not to fall asleep inadvertently.

Spent some time creating a clear second attention against falling asleep and inadvertently exiting. Rolled out. It rolled out, as usual, as if for real, only at the moment of falling to the floor it simply hung in the air, as if falling on an airy blanket. How many hundreds of times I rolled out, but I always have at least a small fraction of the suspicion that I really fall out of bed. A lot of ideas about the use of this position immediately flashed through my head. Immediately quickly drew up a rough plan of action, which included extremely meaningless things. But first, I once again decided to observe space landscapes. I took the goal - space. I was immediately picked up by an unknown force and carried away at breakneck speed. Sight suddenly appears, and I find myself suspended in the vacuum of space in an unknown place. I don't know how real I felt myself, because I had never been in such a place, but, most likely, I felt as if I were there in real life. Prevailing here was vision, everything else quickly ceased to pay attention. I experienced a fantastically pleasant sensation from the galaxy in my field of vision. The unusualness in the perception of vision, apparently, consisted in an unusual focus of the eyes, because in life we rarely look at anything like that, and there everything around required complete parallelism of the eyes. The galaxy was alive, and I remarked to myself that it might be the most beautiful thing I've ever seen. However, it was impossible to stay there for a long time, since there was nothing to concentrate on, because the objects were very far away. He returned to the void and, hovering in a static position, created strong vibrations. For some time I enjoyed this unusual sensation. It was interesting to observe the properties of this phenomenon. When he raised his hands with palms to his face, he felt a strong warm wind flowing from them into his face. There was noise in my ears. When I felt my head with my hands, it seemed that I was touching a bare brain, but there was no pain.

Having enjoyed this state a little, he rushed in an unknown direction. After a short flight, I was thrown out in my room. This time everything in it absolutely corresponded to reality, although such a task was not set. Nothing interested me here, and as if in real life I went through the doors to other rooms. I didn't have to look for adventures for a long time, because in another room I found my mother and brother, whom I had not seen for a long time. I talked to them a little about nothing, only in order to hear their voices, and just looked at them. It was a real gift for me. But he forgot a little and with great difficulty regained control over the state, by the notorious fall upside down ...

Skills and Tips

Phase detection

Often there is a problem of phase identification when entering it, especially for beginners.

The practitioner is simply unable to understand whether he is already in the phase or not yet. Moreover, this uncertainty can arise both when the body is lying down, and during actions outside the body. If the practitioner still remains in the body and does not perform any actions, it is really difficult for him to determine whether he is in the phase or not. It suffices to note that there may be no signs of a phase state. Or, conversely, there may be many signs and unusual sensations, but they will not necessarily indicate the onset of the phase.

However, the problem of state uncertainty is always solved by actions. If the practitioner is lying, then in most cases simple separation techniques can play the role of an indicator, although their implementation may be incorrect. You can also perform various techniques (phantom swinging, rotation, observation of images, etc.), which will definitely manifest themselves in the phase.

But if the practitioner stands up and cannot understand where he has stopped, then it should be borne in mind that in the absolute majority of cases he gets up already in the phase, if such doubts have arisen. However, often, relying on the description that in the "everything is like in reality" phase, a beginner can stand up and note that everything is really "like in reality", and at the same time be in it. But even this situation can be corrected with the help of hyperconcentration, which was discussed in the context of retention in the phase. With its help, you can always understand whether you are in the phase or not. However, as a rule, it rarely comes to this technology. Most often, the following signs can be found, indicating a separation in the phase: unusual sensations in the body during movement, extremely "tight" movements, strong physical pull back to the supine position, inconsistencies in the surrounding space, blurry vision or its absence.

Often the problem lies in the fact that when applying direct techniques, the practitioner expects too fast a result and tries to determine whether he or she is in the phase. In general, this is the wrong approach. When using direct techniques, the phase manifests itself clearly, so if the practitioner tries to identify its presence, this is an indicator that the phase is most likely still far away.

Emergency Return. Paralysis

Studies show that in a third of the first time a phase is experienced, a person experiences fear, which causes him to return back to the body. Periodically, even experienced practitioners have situations that require a sharp return to wakefulness. However, making this return is not always easy. Sometimes it seems that this is simply impossible to do.

Returning directly to the body is almost always easy and effortless. It is enough to remember the body, to think about it, as in a matter of moments you are transferred back to the body, wherever you are. True, with such thoughts it is advisable to close your eyes and try not to touch anything. As a rule, these actions are quite enough, and it remains just to stand up in the physical world. But it is possible that when you return to the body, you will suddenly realize that you are not able to control it, because there is a so-called sleep paralysis, sleep stupor. With him, the body seems to be disabled, paralyzed. At this moment, it is impossible to scream, or call someone for help, or lift a finger. Also, in most cases, it is not possible to open the eyes. From the point of view of science, in this case, there is an abrupt, unnatural interruption of the REM phase, as a result of which such paralysis is inevitable. So, my friend, do not be afraid of such a phenomenon in principle.

You spend up to a quarter of the night in such a stupor, but you just sleep at that time. People in the physical world are accustomed to one important rule: if you want to achieve something, do something, but more actively. This rule is not always suitable for some moments related to the phase. Least of all it relates to getting out of it. Yes, sometimes extreme efforts allow you to break through the stupor and start moving, but more often than not, any effort drives you even more into immobility. That is, more activity - deeper paralysis.

Naturally, against the background of the unusual situation and deliberate return, which, as a rule, is associated with fear, the depth of the phase state can greatly increase. As a result - even more action and even more fear. And even more paralysis. Such a vicious circle gives a lot of unpleasant sensations and emotions, after which not everyone wants to continue any phase practices until they realize their mistakes. And the point is again only in them, as I hope you have already understood.

As a result, ignorance and ignorance of how to act correctly give rise to a widespread opinion that one may not return from the phase at all, therefore it is dangerous to engage in such practices. But it's all about very simple actions that help to avoid so many negative points and false prejudices!

Relaxation

It has been noted more than once: the more activity, the better for depth and phase retention. Accordingly, for exiting the phase, on the contrary, it will be worse. It turns out that in order to get out of the phase, you just need to completely relax, trying to distract yourself from any sensations, actions and thoughts. In parallel with this, you can read a prayer, a mantra or a rhyme, as this allows the mind to quickly distract from the situation. Of course, you need to calm down and try to get rid of fear, which in itself can contribute to paralysis. Periodically, you need to try to move your finger to understand whether the effect of relaxation has begun or not.

Concentration on the finger

In this case, during paralysis, you should try to move one finger or toe. At first it will not work, but you need to concentrate your thoughts and efforts on this particular action. After a while, the physical finger will be able to move.

Concentration of attention on possible movements

You need to know that the physiology of the process of sleep paralysis, phase and dreams is such that part of our capabilities in them is always associated with the real body. This is the movement of the eyeballs, the movement of the tongue and breathing. If you focus on these processes, they can disinhibit all others, after which the practitioner will gain the ability to move in reality. It is a kind of thread that always connects us with reality.

Reassessment of the situation

Keep in mind that under normal conditions, spontaneous exit from the phase cannot be the norm. As a rule, this turn of events is caused by some kind of fears and prejudices. This is a gross mistake. If it is not possible to disinhibit the body using the techniques described above or you have not used any of them (which is even better), it is more important to think about the fact that at the current moment you have the opportunity to be in the phase and that you can experience a lot of interesting and necessary things in it. Why destroy such an opportunity on your own, being unjustifiably wary of something? Come to your senses, and before it's too late, get out of your body and realize your new possibilities!

Emergency phase exit techniques do not always work. As a rule, against the background of a long lack of sleep, at the beginning or in the middle of a night's sleep, the craving for sleep is so great that it is very difficult to resist such a phenomenon as sleep paralysis. In this regard, a reassessment of the situation is very relevant: in order not to suffer, but to use it. It is also worth adding that sleep paralysis is easily transferred into the phase using indirect techniques.

Buddy, knowing how to get out of paralysis is important not only for practitioners of the phase, since sleep paralysis occurs in about a third of the world's population at least once in a lifetime and without falling into the phase. This usually takes place before or after sleep.

Fighting fear

As it has already become clear, fear in the phase is a very common phenomenon. It can strike at any stage of experience, although, of course, at the very beginning it has much more pronounced features. Personally, I had to suffer because of him in the first experiments at least 20 times. But you do not take such a period as a starting point, since I generally did not understand much what it is. And before you everything is already laid out in its purest form, and there are few reasons for fear. However, its modifications can be very diverse: the feeling that it will not be possible to return to the body (death); anxiety that something will happen to the body; meeting in a phase with something terrible; the occurrence of pain; too bright, hyper-realistic feel. However, only one deep cause of fear dominates - the instinct of self-preservation, which evokes in people an outwardly unreasonable animal feeling of horror that cannot be explained and controlled. This is what makes hefty men, who have seen the world in the real world, get out of there, only realizing what happened.

For a beginner who is overwhelmed by an overwhelming sense of fear that does not allow him to do literally anything, there is only one way to gradually conquer fear. Each time in the phase, you need to try to go one step further than it was in the previous case. For example, for the first time through horror, you need to at least raise your hands, and then lower them again. The second time you need to try to sit down. Third time, get up. In the fourth - to resemble. Then the fear begins to recede sharply, and nothing threatens the actions.

Of course, it makes sense to always think more about the fact that in fact nothing threatens you and all the urges to abruptly return to the body are meaningless in nature. Sooner or later, such thoughts begin to be reflected in the events in the phase, and the person gets frightened less and less. However, if we are talking about a momentary fear due to some incident in the phase, then it is easiest to survive it to the end so that there are no more such precedents. If you avoid adverse events all the time, they will overtake more and more often. So I won't even give you advice on how else you can get out of such situations. Not only that, because all these fears in the phase are nothing but the fears of yourself that are clamped down. By implementing them there, you actually get rid of them here. This, by the way, is one of the applied meanings of the phenomenon. And you'll have little choice but to face most of your fears anyway.

Creation of vision

Usually, vision is present in the phase from the very beginning, especially if image observation and visualization techniques are used to enter it. In some cases, vision appears by itself, in the very first seconds. Sometimes it occurs only during the process of deepening in the phase. But there are cases when vision itself does not appear, or when it needs to be created quickly at all costs. In such cases, it happens that it appears, one has only to think about it, but if this does not happen, a special technique should be used. You need to bring your hands to your eyes at a distance of 10-15 cm and try to see them through the gray mist or darkness in front of your eyes. You need to look very carefully and aggressively at the small details of the palms, trying to see them. In just a few seconds, they will begin to appear, as if due to some kind of film. And after a few seconds, the vision will become clear, and not only the palms, but the entire surrounding space will be in front of the eyes.

But keep in mind: when creating vision, in no case should you open your eyes. Vision will appear by itself and will be indistinguishable from the real. Most likely, the sensation of raised eyelids will occur without lifting them. In the phase, you can close your eyes an infinite number of times, while physically never opening them, since vision is created without it. You can open your eyes only in the deep phase. In the shallow phase, this will bring you back to wakefulness as the eyes can actually open.

Friend, you also need to keep in mind that you need to create vision only when you are completely separated from the body, already being in some place. An attempt to see the hands while flying or hovering in an indefinite space leads to involuntary movement.

Communication with objects

During practice, you will notice that in the process of communicating with animate objects, two problems can arise; the silence of these objects or your return back to the physical body. In view of the fact that many applied areas of using the phase are associated with contacts pursuing one goal or another, it is necessary to understand how to behave with people correctly in order to avoid problems. Firstly, during communication, you must follow the elementary rules of retention so that a foul does not happen. For example, look at the details of a person's face or clothes. During communication, you can rub your hands all the time or hold strong vibrations. The bottom line is not to forget about this and much more, carried away by the information received, as is often the case.

But an even more difficult task is to overcome the inadequacy or silence of the living objects of the phase. The problem is that in this case everything is decided not by some specific actions with hands or feet, but by actions of an internal nature. In most cases, the subject's speech is blocked by the inner tension of the practitioner himself. Sometimes the problem is due to the expectation that the object will not be able to talk in phase. That is, the problem is in you, and not in the object, as it may seem.

What can be done here... Remember, you need to treat objects as calmly as possible. Do not try to yell or hit the object in an attempt to get words out of it. It is much more effective to handle him gently, without trying to put pressure on him in any way. It is important not to peer into the subject's lips while waiting for the sounds to be made, or even better, to turn away altogether if nothing else helps.

If it is not possible to talk to the object at the current moment, it will turn out later. Therefore, it is necessary from attempt to attempt to try in different ways to establish a dialogue. As a rule, after the first successes, a kind of turning point occurs, and such a problem no longer arises. The method of communication itself is the same as in everyday life. It is not necessary to use telepathy, it is enough just to express yourself with the help of words, saying them out loud. Try not to create problems for yourself in this.

Reading text

You can read in the phase. But it must be borne in mind that such a reading is fraught with a number of difficulties. For example, small text in the phase is often simply unreadable, since the effect of hyperconcentration can distort it when looking closely. This problem is solved in only one way: you should resort to text sources of information with a large font size. Thus, the text of an ordinary book is often blurry if you start looking at it, but a large title on the cover of the same book can be easily read, since this size is convenient for quick reading without looking.

However, another problem may be that the text turns out to be readable, but at the same time it is completely meaningless, like a set of words or even letters. In this case, it is worth trying to solve the problem by flipping through the pages in search of a normal text, if it is a book or a newspaper. It is also possible to find another instance or recreate it using object finding techniques.

While reading, do not forget about retention techniques, as you can weaken your attention, being distracted by the information received, or simply relax, which usually ends in a foul. In general, this applies to almost all actions in the phase, but many people think that reading can hold, but it is not.

vibrations

Very often, the phase is accompanied by one unusual sensation that cannot be forgotten and which can be successfully used to enter the phase, deepen it, and hold it. It feels difficult to describe it more precisely than "the passage through the whole body of a strong current that does not cause pain." In this case, a feeling of compression of the body, its strong tingling, numbness is possible. Most often, it feels more like a high-frequency vibration of the body, which is why the concept of "vibration" arose.

If you want to understand whether you experienced vibrations or not, there is a good way to answer this question: if there were vibrations, then there will be no doubt that they were exactly them. In all other cases, when doubt and uncertainty are present, there was definitely no vibration. When you face it, you will understand what I mean.

Moreover, if the vibrations have been experienced at least once, remembering these sensations helps very well when using indirect techniques, as one of them. Vibrations are created, maintained and amplified by the tension of the brain or the non-muscular tension of the body. Also, for vibrations to arise, it is often enough just to think about them. At the first experience of them, it is worth experimenting with them for a while, rolling them over the body, strengthening and calming. This will help them to remember and be easier to reproduce in the future.

But one should not think that the presence of vibrations is a necessary condition for being in the phase. Many beginners, having inattentively read various literature, often strive not for a phase, but for vibrations, after which it supposedly should follow. This is the wrong approach. Yes, there are certain techniques that allow you to get into the phase through the creation of vibrations, but in all other cases they are completely optional, and they may never exist at all. This is completely optional, but useful.

Techniques for moving through objects

It has already been noted more than once, my friend, that due to certain laws of the phase in its deepened state, the properties of the surrounding space become very similar to the properties of the physical world. However, sometimes you may need to go through a wall to take a short cut, move, or avoid something. To do this, there are two main options. It usually takes several attempts to master any of them, but some difficulties may arise at the beginning of the practice.

Rapid defocused penetration

To do this, you need to quickly step, jump or run up to the wall, creating in yourself a strong, vivid desire to penetrate it. At this point, you can not peer at the wall. It is desirable that the vision be defocused or directed in the opposite direction altogether. Among other things, you don't need to hold or consider anything from the surrounding space, so as not to linger in this way.

closed eye technique

This technique is a little easier. As you approach the wall, you need to close your eyes and focus on the desire to pass through it. At the same time, one must imagine that there is no wall or that it is transparent, sandy, jelly-like, in general, passable. If there is resistance to the plane, it is necessary to push through it, continuing the same mental concentration. After some attempts, this will be enough.

Flight in phase

Many perceive the phase as the only opportunity to experience the sensations of flight. But not everyone understands in advance that in the deep phase this can be very difficult to do. In order to fly while in the phase, you need to remember how it is done in a dream and then reproduce the same internal actions. There is no need to stress or speak. Although flying with your eyes closed is many times easier, it is better not to do this, as it is possible to move to a place not originally planned.

Even if the flight fails, you can jump from any hill. At this point, it is easy to take control of the fall and turn it into a controlled flight. However, jumping from windows and from any hills is worth it only if you have experience, since a beginner cannot always recognize whether he is in a phase or in reality. Theoretically, this creates a danger of actually falling out of the window. Usually people laugh at this, but I always have to repeat it. There is another option to take off - try to stay in the air while jumping up. This is done in such a way that, having jumped, you are struggling to freeze at the highest point or continue flying even higher. If not from the first, then from the fourth or fifth jump it succeeds.

Superpowers in phase

As already noted, despite the realism of the perception of the space of the phase, it does not limit a person in the ability to survive and do anything. Only he can limit himself out of habit. It is important to remember and understand this: in the phase everything is done simply, not according to the laws of the physical world. For example, if you need to get somewhere, even if it is very far away, you can teleport or, in other words, fly over. If you need some object that is located in another part of the large room, it is not at all necessary to go after it, since it can be attracted with a glance. This is the freedom of action, not limited by habits.

To master such unusual abilities, as a rule, it takes only a few phases to devote to their development. It is almost mandatory to learn how to fly and pass through walls, as the lack of such skills will often affect the experience. You can also learn telekinesis (remote movement of objects), pyrokinesis (set fire to objects with your eyes), telepathy (mind reading) and transformations. Of course, this list can be continued, based on personal needs.

To learn telekinesis, you need to focus your eyes on any object in the full-fledged phase and try to pull it towards you or move it away from you. This must be done with the utmost will. No specific external action is required. The knowledge of how to develop such skills is inherent in any person. If not the first time, then after several attempts, the objects will definitely begin to obey the look and intention. Once you feel how to do it, gaining control over this ability, you can always use it in the phase to increase the comfort of the experience or to carry out some tricks in it.

If you want to learn how to set fire to the surrounding objects with your eyes in the phase, you should, just as in the case of telekinesis, start peering at the necessary objects, strongly wanting to heat them up and set them on fire. Perhaps not the first time, but over time, the object will indeed, after being distorted, light up, darken and smoke.

If you want to develop telepathy skills in the phase, you need to peer into animated objects, while simultaneously listening to the surrounding and internal sounds with the intention of hearing the thoughts of the objects. Even experienced practitioners develop this ability with some difficulties, but when it does develop, it greatly simplifies communication with people in the phase. The most amazing thing is that, having such a skill, one can learn to hear the thoughts of not only people, but also animals and even any inanimate objects in the space of the phase. Yes, that's right - any. However, you should not take what you heard too seriously, as this is just one of the manifestations of the peculiarity of the phase. The accuracy of the information received is a separate topic for discussion.

Also in the phase you can turn things into each other. To do this, you need to focus on the object and imagine another in its place. Gradually, distorting and blurring, the space will obey your will. It is also worth noting the following: if you intend to transform yourself into something, you need to use transfer techniques in which attention is not focused on the desired object, but on the form that you want to give yourself. In this case, again, there are no restrictions, except for your own courage and imagination. You can feel like a butterfly, or you can feel like a dinosaur. It can be a bird, or it can be a worm. You can turn into a child or even change gender. And all this is not just some external changes, but real transformations from the inside and outside. If the practitioner becomes a butterfly, then he has a feeling of wings, many legs and an unusual body. At the same time, he will feel how to manage all this, as if a section appeared in his brain that is responsible for such movements. And this is only the most superficial description of experiences that, in their essence, hardly fit into the usual understanding of the world. It is not for nothing that one of my students often uses the expression that the most amazing thing about the phase is not that you can have sex with any woman in it, but that you yourself can become a woman. It is clear that this means not only the external image, but also the corresponding views on life.

Pain in phase

Of course, friend, along with positive impressions and sensations with the same degree of realism and reliability, opposite sensations may appear in the phase, which may not bring pleasant memories at all. This is easy to check if you approach the wall in the deep phase and hit it with all your might with your fist. The pain will be almost the same as if everything happened in reality. Or even more. Some part of the actions in the phase will inevitably cause pain, so you need to know how to avoid them. To do this, it is necessary during the action to concentrate on the internal confidence that pain will not arise. You can start with the same experiment with the wall: suggesting to yourself that there is no pain, hit it with your fist until pain, even with the strongest blows, does not occur. If you conduct such an experiment at least once, achieving a result will never again require the same efforts. As a rule, it will be enough to think about it and reproduce the desired inner mood.

Exploring possibilities and sensations

Friend, when you start practicing phase experiences, you should not immediately rush in the direction of one thing if the goal is to have a long-term practice. It will be much better to explore this world and everything in it from the very beginning. This will help to feel it better, to know it, which means it is easier to enter into it and apply it.

As in reality, you need to start with the knowledge of what will be revealed to you in the first place. At first, you should simply enjoy the very fact of being in the phase, all the details of this world and their functions, including the most insignificant ones. At first, the practitioner should simply wander around the phase in the place where he will be, looking at everything that catches his eye. If you have a ball in your hands, you can roll it to make sure that the laws of physics apply. If it's a marker, draw it on the wall, etc. The most curious thing is that you don't have to think about it. That's what you'll be doing there the first time anyway. Simple things in this world look completely different when you realize that this cannot be.

In addition, one should try to fully sharpen all possible feelings in the phase in order to fully understand how unusual the phase is in its realism. It is necessary to experience movement: walk, run, jump, take off, fall, swim. Check for pain by hitting the wall with your fist. To test the taste sensations, the easiest way is to go to the refrigerator and try to eat everything you can from it, not forgetting to smell it at the same time. It is also worth trying to go through walls, move around, create objects, etc. All these actions will be very interesting in themselves. Only when they are understood and known, we can assume that the practitioner has an idea about the phase, that it surpasses the physical world in its colors.

The most correct position

From the very beginning, it must be remembered that the condition for the only true way of implementing the practice without unnecessary loss of time is a pragmatic and rational position regarding the nature and possibilities of the phase phenomenon. As a rule, most of the information about the phase that a person gleaned from various sources is the result of a delusion that becomes apparent after the very first real entrances into the phase and experiments carried out in it. That is why it makes sense to start the practice from scratch and profess only one principle: everything is only taken into account until it is confirmed by experience, and only personal experience, and not the experience of acquaintances, book authors, teachers, authors of blog posts and on forums. It would seem that this is a common truth that is clear to everyone, but it only seems. In fact, everyone is immersed in such a myriad of unconfirmed theories and views that it's even scary to think about it. Sometimes it seems that people only consist of this. And this applies, of course, not only to the phase, but to the whole life. Never forget that it is natural for a person to err and to pass on his delusions to others. As a result, many simply paradoxical tales about the phase phenomenon began to be a priori perceived as true. One should not deny everything that is described in the esoteric literature. Perhaps something can be gleaned from it, but you definitely should not take everything written as the ultimate truth. Once again I note: the first instance is you yourself, your experience.

As you know, for a house to stand strong, you need a good foundation. The only option for the practitioner of the phase is to create a good foundation - this initially refers to the phenomenon as mundane as possible, more from a scientific point of view, denying any supernatural phenomena. This approach to business will not allow you to go the wrong way. And on a solid foundation, everyone has the right to build their own truth and their own world. No one has the right to tell you here. Build then whatever you like, but do not forget that all this can collapse or stay on a frail hope until the end of days, if you initially make significant theoretical mistakes. I'm not just talking about this. One day my world collapsed. I got out of the abyss only because I saw the phenomenon from the other side.

Analysis

Buddy, if you want to achieve maximum results, you cannot do without independent intellectual efforts. Here, my recommendations alone are not enough . Remember , as long as all issues are resolved by searching for answers in various sources, no significant progress should be expected. Many things can not be described and explained by anyone. Always a lot of moments remains at the personal discretion and understanding. Finding answers to all questions is simply impossible. Moreover, the search for sources itself sometimes slows down progress very much, because the student-practitioner has to be distracted by tedious reading or talking. Other people may be mistaken, so in no case should there be any unconditional authorities and unattainable ideals. Everything and everyone must be treated initially with a grain of salt. To solve a question, you need to turn on your own thinking more often, and not try to find the answer somewhere. Given that this book contains all the most important topics and questions regarding the phase, it will be quite enough to begin an independent analysis of the phenomenon.

For example, if you encounter some incomprehensible phenomenon or problem while performing techniques for entering the phase or while already in it, first of all you should try to understand its cause on your own. And this is how it should be done every time. You have to rely only on yourself. If you always look for answers outside your own mind, there is a chance to stumble upon a false opinion and adopt it (and even worse - dependence on someone else's shoulder is generally a dead end).

I wouldn't touch this issue if it weren't so relevant. Many stubbornly refuse to analyze their successes and failures, but instead open a variety of books, often contradictory, and extract information from there that they don't even bother to check. This, as a rule, leads to the multiplication of delusions. In my life, I once met a practitioner of the phase who was engaged in it twice as much as I did in time, although several times less in quantitative terms. So, due to the fact that he tried to find the answer to each of his questions in different books, as if afraid to take responsibility for himself or deifying these authors, over decades of practice, he remained exactly where he started. And this is a fairly typical situation. Don't make such mistakes. Everything great is always done from oneself.

Ideal Conditions

Techniques for entering the phase are associated with a special kind of work with the brain, so you need to create such comfortable conditions that the brain reacts as little as possible to external stimuli. Preferably not too cold or too hot. If the room where the techniques are performed is very bright, it is recommended to shield the eyes from bright light. A special soft sleep mask is well suited for this. Since it does not always hold up well, especially during a restless dream in the morning, you can use the usual thick dark-colored hat, pulling it over your eyes. Of course, all this will not be needed if there are thick curtains on the windows that create the effect of twilight in the room. Frequent irritants are noise, so you need to think about soundproofing in advance. It is usually enough to turn off the sound of the phone, close the doors and windows. If this does not help or the environment is too noisy, you can use ordinary earplugs. It is not superfluous to warn others so that you are not disturbed. It is desirable that there is no one else on the bed where you will do the techniques. Most often, pets interfere in this case, so they should be fed in advance and left outside the room where you are going to practice. No wonder I like to call cats the main "astral terrorists". You can wake up in the morning and not move, hoping for excellent trips in the phase, but the cat knows that you are no longer sleeping, but it is time to open the refrigerator. Such a mess will cause an innocent animal to disturb you and run into trouble. Therefore, it is better to take care of such things in advance.

Like-minded people

Never forget that there is great benefit in discussing your own and others' experiences with other practitioners. This leads to the exchange of information, the acquisition of new knowledge and mutual assistance in solving certain problems and issues. Of course, personal communication has the greatest effect. It is desirable to meet like-minded people more often in reality. The phase is one of the most unusual experiences, and it is always interesting how others describe their feelings, how they do it. Since this topic is still very poorly covered in society, it is possible that there will be problems with finding interlocutors. This can be solved by spreading information about your practice, which will certainly be of interest to someone around you. It is even better to pass on educational literature to friends, at least the same book.

Diary

A friend will greatly help in learning the phase of keeping your own diary. It allows not only to clearly fix what happened, but also to be aware of it. Moreover, if kept properly, a diary helps develop the ability to analyze events in a phase, which immediately raises the quality of experience to a completely different level, as we have already discussed. It allows you to overcome the chaos of practice, turning it into a structured and clear study. If your personal practice does not turn into your personal research, then you will never achieve anything significant. Again, this is not just about the phase. The diary itself should contain many indicators so that, if necessary, statistical studies can be carried out to identify some patterns. The diary must indicate the date and time of day (1). Next, you should give a detailed description of entering the phase and experiences in it (2), list the mistakes made (3), draw up an action plan for the next phase (4). These four points should always be clearly separated and understood. Moreover, when describing your experience, pay more attention to technical details, rather than describing beauty and sensations. It makes sense for a beginner to write down information even about unsuccessful attempts to get into the phase. Then only successful phase experiences can be noted.

Case Study

May, 2001
Immediately after lunch, I decided to enter the phase in a direct way, for which I began to try to use the dotting technique (concentration of attention on different parts of the body). However, during relaxation, I encountered difficulties: I could not calm my thoughts that were carried away by other things. I had difficulty concentrating on the task. Did a relaxation. Then doted again for about 20 minutes, but nothing worked, although slight vibrations appeared from time to time. But more and more I wanted to sleep. At one moment, the consciousness turned off, but instantly it woke up (as it seemed to me, it lasted no more than a minute, which was proved by hours after returning to the body) under the influence of a preliminary intention not to sleep, after which a feeling of cheerfulness suddenly appeared, and I was already absorbed by the vibrations that from such a jump in physiological states they themselves appeared. I easily managed to strengthen them. Then rolled out. But the vibrations immediately began to weaken, and I was returned to the body. Then it began to separate again, by simply crawling out. With

great effort, I managed to do it. And I hovered in an indefinite space and with vague sensations. I experienced a strong sense of discomfort during the separation, which persuaded me to stop this attempt, but I remembered that this sometimes happens and always disappears when immersed in a more stable phase. To deepen the phase, this time I decided to use the sensation of flight. It worked, and I really enjoyed the process. The flight, for some unknown reason, did not lead me to the deepest phase, so for further diving I began to fall headfirst. As he moved and deepened, he experienced slight anxiety, which was on the verge of fear, but at first he controlled it. At a certain moment, I realized that I was in such a deep state, in which I had never been before. This increased the anxiety. For the sake of the experiment continued to rush down. Thoughts began to appear about the impossibility of returning to the body from such a depth. Vision was either there or not, because I was only concerned with my sensations, but not with what could be seen around. When vision appeared, what I saw cannot be described in words, it was so unusual, vague and realistic, as if I see it with some other organ of vision, incomparably more developed. I did not feel the body (neither real nor phantom). For the first time in my life, I physically felt my thoughts: when I thought about something, I began to move arbitrarily in space, and I clearly felt that the reason for this movement was my thoughts; my brain seemed to move with thoughts (I experienced this feeling for the first time, so I can't say how real I experienced it, if at all it is possible to experience it in a normal state, but the feeling was very real). Realizing a very deep position in the phase, I decided to get out of there, worried for my life. It is easy to assume that getting out was, to put it mildly, not very easy. He began to feel fear. I could not enter the body in any way, gain control over it. I was finally able to feel it, but it was like it wasn't mine. Even concentrating on my big toe didn't help me, which was hard to expect. Relaxation, instead of taking you out of the state, deepened. Then I was completely at a loss: what always helped did not help, and there were no other effective ways. After many desperate attempts, I finally managed to enter the body. It happened simply by trying to move something and concentrating on breathing.

Chapter Four

Applied value

Well, dear friend, it's time to talk about what will be the main motivation for you in mastering the technologies described in this book. If you knew how wonderful this state is in its nature, you would not care about its applied significance. In any case, the first time. This in itself is the most amazing thing possible. But you still may not have time to understand or experience it, so at the beginning of your path some applied side will move you, and I tried to exhaustively describe everything related to this to you. All this will be especially useful to those who already know how to take their consciousness beyond the body. The fact is that few people understand the true scope of the phenomenon. That is why people often waste their amazing experiences on insignificant things or try in vain to get something from them that is only a theory that no one has proven in practice.

Everything described below is the real foundation for your practice. All this, despite the fantastic nature of some sections, is available to everyone, regardless of worldview.

Meetings and travel

Trips

Tell me what can make it possible to be anywhere you can think of? What can make it possible to meet with anyone who only ever existed or did not even exist? And all this can be known without getting off the bed, quickly, in the whole reality of experiences and without any harm to health. Agree, it is impossible to believe in it if you do not know about the existence of the phase. But it is she who allows, without taking the soft spot off the sofa, to be in any situation, you just want to.

Be sure, if you want to go to some place, you will find yourself in it, as if in full reality, even if you have never been there. Getting to well-known places, you absolutely can not find any differences from reality. And most importantly, everything will be very real, and you can experience the same feelings that you would experience if you were actually present in this place, whether it be a feeling of delight from the high Chomolungma or cold and blinding brightness at the North Pole.

Buddy, have you always dreamed of flying into space? There is nothing easier. The Travel Techniques section details how you can get to absolutely any place in the universe. It doesn't matter the distance or anything else. Have you looked at photographs of galaxies and stars many times, but did not even think that such beauty can be seen almost live from any distance? I didn't think so either, but I have had a different opinion for a long time, and more than once I had to get incredible pleasure from observing various kinds of cosmic objects and events. This is truly amazing!

You do not have the money or the opportunity to finally see the great Egyptian pyramids live? Have you ever dreamed of being at the very top of the pyramid of Cheops or riding the Sphinx? No? Now you can dream about anything and not be afraid that it will never come true. Now nothing can stop you from fulfilling any, even the most crazy dream. And seeing the pyramids is even more than simple, and you can come up with something much more interesting and inaccessible in the physical world.

In the phase, you can enjoy the landscape of any kind, starting with the usual mountain range and ending with the landscape of Mars in the morning during sunrise. Or maybe you have lived all your life in a cold northern country - and only now you can soak up the shores of a small island in the Indian Ocean? Once again I say: no problem - although, of course, you first need to get some skills, but it's not difficult.

Maybe you have been interested in history all your life, and you were attracted by the events of bygone days? Of course, then it will be interesting to see medieval Paris, Ancient Rome or Constantinople. Maybe it will be interesting for you to get into the era of the first settlers who founded the future US superpower? There are no problems, because time does not exist in the phase. It is a common thing when different times and cultures are intertwined in it. You can visit not only the past, but also the future, and such a journey can bring you really useful information. Have you always been stunned by the movie "Jurassic Park", where in the form of a well-realized film illusion, the cherished dream of many people was realized - to see living dinosaurs? With its realism, this film allows you to temporarily forget that this is a movie. But in the phase you can not only meet with a mastodon, a pterodactyl and have a good look at them, but you can even touch and feed them with certain settings. I know a man who decided to do out-of-body travel just because of the opportunity. And he was not disappointed, having met, as if alive, dinosaurs, which he had never dreamed of before. And this is not only fun for students who have completely lost their heads from the possibilities of the phase, but for adults and even the elderly.

Meetings

Naturally, dreams of no lesser scale can be realized by meeting various people in the phase, and not necessarily those who have ever been seen alive. It is possible to find any person about whose existence at least something is known, even if only a name. Imagine what space for fantasy this state of affairs opens up! You can meet absolutely any historical figure without any restrictions. Everything is available there, from Confucius, Tutankhamen I, Cleopatra, Napoleon, etc.

These opportunities will be of particular interest to ardent admirers or fans of any famous figures in cinema, sports and music. It suffices here to give an example of Elvis Presley. No one will ever accurately calculate the number of his fans around the globe, although he has long been gone from us. It is still popular and one of the most frequently invoked in séances, which are often held just for its sake. The phase allows anyone to meet him, and at the same time the event will be like in reality. Many Elvis fans do not even dream of such an opportunity, and this is not a joke at all. You can meet with any of the famous people, but also with someone from your environment and relatives, both living and dead. In general, you can meet any dear person. There is only one limitation in this area. It is even difficult to call it a limitation, because it is often limitless, especially for creative people. This is your wish. Everything in the phase is limited only by him. If you have a poor imagination, then you still have some dreams - so take care of their implementation. Finally it's possible!

At this stage in the development of human civilization, nothing can compare with the phase in many respects.

No computer or medical device will give you so many positive results.

creative development

I am sure that any creative person who reads this book has more than once come up with the idea of the widest possibilities for using this phenomenon for cultural and creative purposes. Indeed, it is difficult to imagine any boundaries in this direction. In addition to the lack of a limit from a technical point of view, there are no boundaries in the nature of creativity. And the artist, and the musician, and the sculptor, and the designer - everyone will be able to use the practice of the phase for their own purposes. Moreover, the application can be in two main and most important areas: firstly, modeling the product of creativity and, secondly, the path to an unlimited source of new sensations, feelings and experiences that move a person to new fantasies and creations. For the latter, a simple practice of these experiences is sufficient. It's really enough to get access to the gushing source of fantasy. I am silent about the search for an object of creativity in the phase in order to realize it in reality.

The use of the phase for modeling a product of creativity is obvious, because in this state it is possible to create absolutely everything. The artist will be able to create a picture that he is just about to paint or has already partially painted. This gives him the opportunity to evaluate the result in advance and make any changes, if necessary. Or he can look through all the pictures he is going to paint and choose the most desirable one for work. In addition, he can simultaneously compare all the pictures he has ever seen, since the space of the phase will easily reproduce them for him in the smallest detail.

This feature of the phase will be very useful for musicians, because it allows you to create musical masterpieces of any complexity, including those with the use of an orchestra and a choir, the actions of which can be easily and naturally controlled without thinking about how difficult it is to do this or that, or about not to overwork people who must obey your every will. Also, you don't have to think about whether the orchestra, for example, can immediately reproduce the sounds the way you want, because the sound will always correspond to the desires. Naturally, for this you first need to master the phase control, but is this really an obstacle?

A sculptor or architect can easily create any creation and examine it in detail, thus being able to find out any weaknesses in advance. It makes no sense to describe how a representative of one or another type of creativity can use the properties of the phase; such people can guess about it on their own. Undoubtedly, each of them can find something for themselves there. It should also be noted that created products in this state do not disappear into nowhere. That is, you will not need to worry about reproducing an object that has already been created in previous phases. It is stored there forever, and you can always find it. In other words, you can store any information there in perfect accuracy.

The only thing a creative person can worry about is recreating in reality those brilliant masterpieces that he can easily create in the phase. The fact is that the space of the phase is much more powerful than our consciousness, that is, in reality, we have much less abilities. However, there will always be an opportunity to get back into the phase and refine the details. In fact, everything is limited only by our primitive memory, which is not able to remember a large amount of information.

Even I, my friend, a person far from musical creativity, was able to easily create truly brilliant musical masterpieces of various genres in the phase, from the reproduction of which I received incredible pleasure and subsequently only regretted that I could not and did not have the knowledge and opportunities for recreating them in reality.

sports improvement

In many areas of human activity, the skill of any complex physical movements is of great importance, on which everything sometimes depends. However, motor skills play a major role in most sports, for example, in martial arts, from wrestling to fencing, gymnastics, weightlifting, figure skating, etc. In many ways, these sports consist in bringing some movements to automatism. To do this, gymnasts perform somersaults or other elements dozens of times during training, wrestlers polish the same throw for months.

For such people, there is another additional movement training that can be done in the phase. It may seem to some that this does not make sense, but during movements in the phase, the same action occurs in the brain as during wakefulness, only the nerve signal is not sent to the muscles. Based on this, any trained movement in the phase will be practically trained in the same way in real life. This feature allows you to expand your workouts or even replace them during injuries or inability to train for any other reason. Of course, you will never become an Olympic champion by training in this way, but it is still very effective, which I have verified in my experience.

It just so happened that fans of martial arts are no less addicted to the phase. It is for this reason that you often meet people who either work out some actions in the phase or simulate sparring with strong opponents. But it is even more interesting to find famous personalities for the master class in the phase. Steven Sigal , Jackie Chan and, of course, Bruce Lee are especially popular here . Well, do not forget one more interesting detail: with the technologies for obtaining information, which are also described in this book, you, my friend, will be able to find out exactly how you train, what technologies and opportunities to use to improve and succeed in your sport. If you, of course, do it, which I sincerely hope.

New life for the disabled

For most people, this practice is still entertainment or, at best, a way of self-development. But for people with disabilities, it can acquire a completely different, simply revolutionary meaning. For the disabled, the space of the phase sometimes turns out to be the only place where they can feel not only complete, but also much freer and even more capable than healthy people in the everyday physical world.

Suppose a person who has lost his sight will see again in the phase, and it will be better than in reality. And the immobilized will be able not only to walk and run, but also to fly. He who has lost his hearing will regain the ability to hear the murmur of the stream and the singing of birds. And this is only the most general description of the possibilities that the phase provides. In fact, the practice of the phase for a disabled person is an opportunity to discover a new, incomparable world, against the background of those simple things that healthy people do not even notice, but they are very important for a person (just walk, just see, for example) . Against the backdrop of a deprived everyday life, for many of them this may be the only way to receive any additional emotions.

There are some nuances that should be understood in advance. For example, if a person is blind from birth, then there is no guarantee that in the phase he will acquire the same vision as in healthy people. However, this issue has not been fully studied, and such people just need to train on their own, still trying to see, since it is theoretically possible.

Also, limited capabilities in some cases may adversely affect the practice of phase states. For example, it is more difficult for those who are blind to catch intermediate states between sleep and wakefulness due to the fact that their full awakening, unlike the awakening of the sighted, can occur without opening their eyes, against the background of the perception of surrounding sounds. However, this is not a problem, as they have many other positive factors for practice that other people lack.

In any case, this area of application of the phase state requires further study and additions. It deserves serious attention, as it is an effective tool for the rehabilitation of disabled people, unique in terms of experience. For many years now, I have been promoting certain projects in this direction and educating disabled people for free. One of my goals in life is to create a large-scale international structure that will only deal with the issue of educating disabled people and bringing them information about the practice of the phase.

Bad computer games

Mankind has come up with many ways of entertainment and has always given this issue one of the priorities in life. Many psychologists believe that all human actions are ultimately driven by the desire to have fun, and entertainment is, in many ways, that's why it's so important. This allows you to partly forget the difficulties of life and immerse yourself in the intriguing sensations of the most diverse types. Someone likes to travel, someone likes to go to the cinema or just watch TV at home, someone likes to play football or go shopping, etc. In this area, humanity has reached a high diversity, unusual for any other creatures on the planet. No one will argue that for most males, computer games occupy one of the most important places in the field of entertainment and recreation. The digital world really conquers the inquisitive male mind with diversity and versatility. There we can find an infinite number of things that have no right to exist in reality. There you can feel like anyone, from a soldier to a god. This is a really powerful distraction from the gray reality.
But is this the limit of possibilities with this approach? Is the computer world really that exciting, or does it seem that way because you can't compare it to anything else? Is it possible to experience the sensations of movement or any movement in space while being in the process of a computer game ? Can you touch anything in the computer world? Nothing but keys or a mouse. Only the actual simulation of interaction with objects is created. Is there at least one person who managed to taste the sensations of food while in the virtual world? Most people are sure that it is impossible to get such sensations in any other way than by actually eating food, and this is far from being the case. Maybe virtual

digital worlds are not as good as they seem? All computer reality is just watching a flat small screen and pushing buttons. The only real senses involved are hearing and partially sight. All other sensations are fully present in the gray everyday life. Playing computer games is in fact nothing more than just peeping through a narrow gap for an interesting digital dimension, and at the same time we completely remain in our familiar world.

But traveling in phase space is an order of magnitude superior not only to virtuality, but even to the physical world, if we talk about possible perceptions and their brightness. There you can have a tasty meal, and shoot from weapons, and have a close chat with any girl, and find yourself in outer space. In this case, everything will be indistinguishable from reality. Outside the physical body , it is possible not only to feel all the familiar sensations, but also to know those that everyday life will never allow you to know (for example, feel like an insect, fly in space, go through a wall, transform something, etc.). It is not for nothing that many consider being in this world (phase space) an opportunity to more fully experience their existence. We can say that this occupation no longer competes with the computer world, but with real life.

To understand how much more realistic the experience of any actions in the phase is than similar ones in the computer world, it is enough to know the reaction of people who are familiar with both. Even any professional gamer with extensive experience, being out of the body for the first time, cannot calm down from the experience for a very long time: it shocks the human mind so much. Even such a sophisticated mind in entertainment can be shocked. And in general, any entry into this parallel world at the initial stages of practice is very emotionally perceived by all people.

After all of the above, the idea of the possibility of mass use of the practice of the phase, including as an alternative to computer games, cannot but appear. In any case, it can become a completely new means of entertainment, competing with all the most famous and popular methods. Moreover, it is not difficult to assume that, under certain conditions, this can produce a real revolution in this direction. It is one thing to look at the screen of a flat monitor and immerse yourself in certain worlds with a minimum number of feelings, it is another thing to completely, with all your being, go into an even more perfect, intelligent and boundless world, the experiences of which are often no less real than our everyday life. It does not require absolutely no equipment or devices, you do not need to spend money on it. It is at the same time more accessible, more extensive and more interesting than the computer, virtual world. Moreover, such a practice implies powerful personal growth.

Of course, it is impossible to assert that the practice of the phase is a 100% alternative to the computer, but, in any case, this is how it happens in many aspects of the field of entertainment, and we will talk about processing and receiving information in the phase separately. Among other things, in search of new and unusual sensations, people do not always come to the computer. Unfortunately, they often find drugs. Maybe this world gives some unusual experiences, but from the outside it is clear that the consequences of this bring too many troubles and problems. And from this point of view, the practice of the phase will be an ideal field for searching for those very new sensations.

The only way to meet the deceased

Using the technologies of finding objects in the phase, you will be able to meet any person in it, alive or not. This is a separate broad topic, but most of it in the applied sense is occupied by the opportunity to meet with a deceased relative, and not with some famous historical figure, for example. It is clear, dear friend, for us the greatest grief is death. Your death in the future and loved ones in the present. This is natural, since no one has yet managed to avoid biological death. We are used to losing forever and we discard any thoughts about continuing communication as stupid, paradoxical and fantastic. Someone believes in resurrection and that sometimes souls can come from the afterlife, but due to the lack of any specific techniques that could make it available to everyone, nothing but skepticism among the broad masses comes out of this. . But is it all hopeless? Is it true that each of us believes that the loss is forever? And if there is a specific method of achieving contact with a dead person, then how should we relate to everything else in our life?

So far, no one can say for sure what the phase is for the phenomenon and what its true nature is. But one thing is known: it allows you to apply yourself in various areas of human existence, including meeting with dead people. It is possible, tested and has a step by step technical description. It can be said without exaggeration that mankind loses a lot by not paying attention to such a completely real possibility of a phase, regardless of whether you are a materialist or an idealist. But after all, this is the only really real opportunity to consciously and directly make contact with a deceased loved one (or not), which sometimes you really want and that seemed completely impossible.

And everyone can experience it for themselves. If you hold this book in your hands, after reading it, you will soon be able to meet again with those whom you no longer hoped to see until the end of your days. Is there anything comparable to this, my friend?

Moreover, the person you meet in the phase will be as real in perception as if you found him in the everyday world. It can be touched. You can talk to him, hear the same timbre of voice. You can hug him. Even the smell... It's not imagination and not some vague image - it can be even brighter than the world that is now in front of you. Of course, I will not talk about the nature of the people we can find there. For some, these are real souls. Some people don't believe in souls as such. You know, my friend, people in the physical world look at the same things in different ways. Will the situation be easier in the phase? Of course not. It is for this reason that it is absolutely not worth dwelling on this moment. The main thing is that it can be done. And more importantly, there's no other way to do it. The algorithm is simple: entering the phase, deepening, finding objects. And then - if only there was enough courage ...

Behavior of the deceased person in the phase

In general, technically, except for fear, there are no difficult obstacles to meet a dead person in the phase. But there are several basic types of his behavior, which I will talk to you separately. Whatever theory of the nature of the phase you are warmest of all, no matter what properties it offers, there are still several characteristic types of behavior of such objects in the phase. All the oddities of the behavior and character of a person encountered in the phase almost always manifest themselves in the very first seconds of communication with him, although situations are not rare when abrupt changes begin to occur only after a while.

Keep in mind that changes in the psychology of the object and the nature of communication during contact are most often characteristic of those cases when a person still does not quite clearly control the phase, making various mistakes that lead to such failures. With solid practical experience and the ability to confidently use phase control techniques, such situations become exceptions rather than rules. So the options are:

• behavior as deceased ;
• behavior as if alive;
• tearfulness and pity;
• cadaveric syndrome;
• aggression;
• unwillingness to communicate;
• the behavior of a stranger;
• absolute inadequacy.

Behavior as deceased

A description of this pattern of behavior cannot be given in exact detail, but it can certainly be characterized by the following: a person realizes that he was once alive, and now he is dead. At the same time, the properties and possibilities of behavior may not correspond to the possibilities of the organism in the physical world, since there is no internal limitation. This is the most common behavior of a deceased person in the phase, which, perhaps, one should always strive to achieve in order to maximize the reliability of the situation. Moreover, with such behavior of the object, the most complete communication actually occurs, the actual continuation of what once took place in the physical world. That is, there is no interruption of the logical chain with the corresponding silences, etc. If we consider the situation from the position of life after death, then one should always strive to achieve precisely this human behavior.

How to interact with a dead person in the phase, if he understands that he is dead? You don't have to think too much about this moment. It is better to act on the basis of the situation, trying not to hurt anything painful and capable of causing negative emotions. Talk about everything as it really is.

Behavior like a living

A person met in the phase, who died in reality, can have all the possible external properties and behavior that we are used to in reality, starting with the same manner of dressing and ending with the usual style of conversational speech. This person can act as if life is still going on and as if you are just meeting him in everyday life. That is, he may not notice and be unaware of the situation, as if life is still supported by the beating of the heart.

Most often, in this situation, the object does not have any special knowledge and capabilities in controlling the phase, and all its actions do not differ in any way from those in the physical world, limited by its laws, which, by and large, no matter what the phase is, does not have a place in it. Faced with this kind of human behavior, you may be quite satisfied with it, as you wish, or maybe not. The fact is that if the object is aware of his position, this can seriously affect his attitude to everything around him, creating unnecessary problems and unnecessary worries for him. If you don't like this behavior for any reason, you can use the contact techniques again, emphasizing that the object does not appear again with the same view of the surrounding space. You can also just tell him about his death, but this is fraught with a number of negative forms of behavior. By and large, with such a psychological appearance, one can quite reasonably communicate in the same way as it once took place during his lifetime. It is in this case that the reaction will be the most adequate and acceptable for you and for him.

Tearfulness and pity

In this case, the deceased person in the phase behaves as if regretting what happened to him in the physical world, which led him to this situation. This is expressed in constant complaints, tears and a reminder of what happened. This behavior is most often manifested in those moments when a little time has passed since the death of a person.

For some, this behavior will be normal and does not require further decision. If this does not suit you, since looking at all this is not very pleasant, then the most correct solution to the problem will be to try to convince the deceased that nothing terrible is happening, everything is fine, because it should be so. In general, you need to apply the typical consolations for such a case. Perhaps they will gain their strength very quickly. This is better than reloading the contact again.

cadaveric syndrome

This possible scenario is the most undesirable and should be avoided using all available methods. If you inadvertently meet a deceased person in this form, you may simply never want to go through all this again, but the reason will lie solely in the incorrect technical performance of the task. The cadaveric syndrome of a deceased person in the phase fully corresponds to its name. Having completed the contact technique, you will find yourself on a date with a corpse, which is most terrible if a person has once died and received severe injuries during this. Cadaverous syndrome can be divided into two main types. Firstly, an ordinary cadaveric syndrome, when a person is immobilized, maybe in a coffin. Secondly, the living corpse syndrome, when a person looks like a dead person (cadaveric spots, a cold body, lack of a pulse, breathing, and even stitches from an autopsy), but at the same time, he can move and contact you quite normally.

As soon as after performing the contact technique you realize that you are in just such a situation, immediately stop this contact, as it can have very deplorable consequences. However, do not think that after this all attempts to interact with dead in the phase will occur in a similar way. You can refute this at the next contact, perhaps right there, without returning to reality.

If you decide to continue contact with a person who does not differ from a corpse, then you need to do this as carefully as possible, trying not to focus on his condition. I cannot fail to note that all these reservations mostly concern meetings with deceased relatives. I know people who deliberately, solely for the sake of curiosity, find corpses there. You don't have to wonder if this is correct or not. One way or another, but such an opportunity also exists, and it can be useful for combating the acute fear of the dead.

Aggression

This kind of psychology of a dead person in the phase, as the name implies, is characterized by aggression caused by a variety of reasons. This can be expressed in attempts to inflict physical harm on you, kill, scare you, threaten you. Each of these points can have the most diverse form, for which there is a very favorable ground in the space of the phase, thanks to its unlimited properties. The reasons for this behavior can be varied. In no case should you consider it normal and you should not try to adapt to it.

The most important thing in contact with an object with such a psychological type of behavior is getting around without physical impact on it. It must be remembered that whatever contact may be, it may be reflected in subsequent interactions, therefore, it is always worth stopping communication if it turns out that not everything is in order. Especially if this is a relative, it is not so easy to psychologically survive his death and another fight with him. If the object is very actively attacking you, immediately apply the movement technique. You can also immediately try to re-establish contact.

Reluctance to communicate

In this case, the deceased person begins to behave very aloofly and without the desire to make contact in communication. It must be said right away that such behavior in the phase is not the prerogative of only the deceased . This problem is very common in almost all cases of communication with animate objects in the phase. This is especially pronounced in the early stages. In practice, it looks like this: when you approach a person, not believing your eyes, happily trying to hug him, you will not only not see the same thing in his eyes, but everything will look as if he sees you for the first time. When you try to ask or explain something, you will not see the typical reaction of a living person. The answer is often one silence. At this point, the deceased often tries to hide his eyes.

The problem is solved by developing the skills of communication with animated objects in the phase. In addition, just a good practical level often helps, at which there are very few such minor flaws.

Stranger Behavior

Now let's consider the case when the deceased will behave quite adequately in terms of communication and interaction, but at the same time will not show signs that he was once familiar with you. A person can be exactly the same as you are used to seeing him, have the same qualities of character and physical data. Perhaps he will know his name, but everything else, especially his story, will have nothing to do with reality. It is quite reasonable to assume that the absence of a real memory in a deceased person will not be an obstacle to communication. And really, does it really matter if you finally saw him again? This is better than nothing, so at first it is unlikely that the thought will arise that the contact was not successful, and the desire to take measures to correct it, because this type of communication allows you to see the same eyes again, hear the same voice, etc.

Maybe the deceased does not need to remember at all what happened to him and where he is? Maybe let him live in his dreams, seeing the whole situation in a different light? Is it really necessary for you to see those torments that can be born in him after realizing the situation? Therefore, before taking measures to achieve more natural conditions of contact, think carefully about their expediency.

If you interact with a person who does not remember the past, then you need to do this in the most natural way, since this is most justified. Just remember: a reminder of what you have experienced can cause unwanted reactions in the deceased , and then you will have to get to know him again and establish communication.

Absolute inadequacy

In some cases, the behavior of a deceased person in the phase is similar to the behavior of a madman, with the most versatile manifestations of this anomaly, ranging from inadequate perception of the surrounding space to the lack of articulate speech and extreme aggressiveness of the object.

Once again, I note that the behavior of deceased people in the phase, especially at the initial stages of mastering it, can very much depend on how the person died, as well as on how exactly you saw all the moments adjacent to this process (funeral, for example). Therefore, if before death a person showed some notes of madness, then they could very easily find a place in the space of the phase.

In this case, of course, it is unlikely to be able to resolve the situation in a positive way and convert the object's inadequate behavior into normal. It is worth immediately using the techniques of re-reaching contact, in which, most likely, such strange behavior will no longer be.

Case Study

October, 2006

Don't eat while watching the news. Today's entire breakfast ended up in the toilet after I vomited from the message that one of my acquaintances, far from the last person in this world, was brutally murdered that night. A couple of weeks ago, he tried to get through to me, but I had no desire to communicate with him at his regular drinking parties. I immediately decided to somehow compensate for this for my mind. Leg. With great difficulty he calmed down and began to concentrate on the phantom swaying of the arm. They did not appear for a long time, but, having appeared, they began to rapidly increase in their amplitude, and after ten minutes, after a slight failure of consciousness, I was able to calmly get out of bed. Deepening was not required, and, closing my eyes, I immediately concentrated on the image of my acquaintance. I was immediately picked up by something and carried in an unknown direction. A few seconds later, I was literally thrown into the kitchen of my friend's apartment. As usual, he sat in an armchair near a table laden with cognac. Didn't pay any attention to me. His appearance was unhealthy: a lot of smudges, bruises, spots, cuts. Although there was almost no blood, because of the hyper-realism, it was scary to look at all this, and I again felt nauseous. As I got closer, he turned to me and sobbed... I tried to ask him what happened, because the news didn't say how it happened. It turned out that his lifestyle was to blame. He started screaming that he wanted to live, that he wouldn't act like this again if he lived again. I apologized for not picking up the phone. I looked at him for the last time. And, contrary to his own commandments, he himself returned to the body. In the evening, his explanation of what happened was confirmed. As for his behavior and appearance, it is clear that it was caused by my emotions. I think if I meet him in a couple of months, he will look and act differently.

Receiving the information

Dear friend, forgive me, but I'm going to take a couple of pages now just to talk to you about theories. This is the rare case when theory will be useful for practice. Let's start with the fact that obtaining knowledge from a phase state implies access to certain information resources. The catch is that these resources are not known to anyone, since there is no clear data. However, we should think about something. Some confidently believe that the whole point is in the information fields to which we have access in the phase. In addition to being fantastic, nothing can be noted in this statement, since indeed the amount of information received makes you believe in anything, if you look directly at practice. Some are adherents of the view that the collective unconscious is to blame for everything, which, however, does not go so far from that very judgment about the information field. Almost from the same area are the mythical Akashic Chronicles and other teachings from the "universal libraries". Not everything can be listed here. Moreover, from the occult directions, the theory that the information received in the phase comes from some beings from other worlds looks quite natural. It is especially easy to think this way when using the technique of animated objects to obtain information, which we will talk about a little later. However, it is worth keeping a sober mind and drawing conclusions solely from practice, and not from books, theories and someone's personal impressions. I remind you that experience is the only measure of truth. One way or another, we cannot ignore the most mundane explanation of this phenomenon, which says that this is a hyper-realistic dissociative state of the brain. In this case, the source of information is the brain itself, and the subconscious comes to the fore. Most modern practitioners still adhere to this particular position, especially since it has the most significant and intelligible explanations.

For example, let's assume that the phase state is just an exceptionally unusual state of the brain and all perception in it is nothing more than an unusual realistic play of its functions. Suppose a practitioner in a phase decides to move to the forest. To do this, he used the technique of closed eyes, as a result of which a forest grew in front of him in a couple of seconds. But what will happen if we realize in detail what a forest is, what it consists of and where it all came from? Buddy, think about it, because in seconds the human brain was able to create a hyper-realistic space that is not inferior to reality, which consists of millions of blades of grass, leaves, hundreds of trees, many sounds. Each blade of grass consists of something, and is not a point, it can be taken, pulled out of the ground and even the root system can be seen. Each leaf consists of living tissue with veins. The bark of the tree has a natural unique pattern. All this, it turns out, was able to create a resource in the brain, and in seconds. Try it, believe that your brain can do it, although sometimes you can't remember the simplest things in your life...

And now the wind has blown in the forest, and millions of leaves and blades of grass, obeying the mathematical model of the distribution of air masses, start undulating. It turns out that a certain resource within us is capable of not only creating millions of details in the right order in just seconds, but also managing each of these details separately. Even if the phase is just a state of the brain, this does not mean the absence of a source of information, because the brain has a huge computing resource, the power of which is almost impossible to realize. It is unlikely that at least one, even the most advanced computer, is capable of this. It turns out that the practitioner has the opportunity to contact this source in the phase. It remains to be seen: how exactly to do this? If we proceed from the fact that the subconsciousness is engaged in the space, its formation and control in the phase, then it turns out that it is with him that you can contact in the phase state. It is quite possible that the subconscious gives us some information signals in everyday life based on the calculations of its huge resource. But we do not hear and do not perceive. This happens because we are accustomed to perceive everything through words, but it is unlikely that the subconscious mind will operate with such a weak tool for exchanging information. Only a phase can allow you to consciously communicate with the subconscious. If all its objects are created and controlled by the subconscious, then they can be used as translators. For example, when talking to a person in the phase, we hear the usual words, while the object itself and its knowledge at that moment are controlled by the subconscious.

Of course, the essence of obtaining information in the phase can hardly be considered a fully proven and unconditional fact. The above is nothing more than a theory. Perhaps completely different resources are involved in this, but this is not so important. The most important thing is that it is known how information can be obtained in the phase.

Ways to get information

There are only three main techniques for obtaining information in the phase, but each of them is very diverse in its essence. These are the technique of animate objects, the technique of inanimate objects, and the technique of plot. Of course, there are some other techniques, but it is hardly worth thinking about them when these three provide everything that any practitioner needs for any purpose.

Animated Object Technique

To implement this technique of obtaining information in the phase, you need to find a person (using the techniques of finding an object) and ask him for the necessary information (simple questions). If the received information is connected with some person, then it is he who must be found in the phase. If the information is not associated with a specific person, then it is possible to create a universal source of information, which must necessarily be associated with wisdom and knowledge. For example, it can be some kind of sage-hermit, a well-known healer in reality, etc. The advantage of the technique: you can easily ask a clarifying question and just as easily check the information received. Lack of technology: many people find it difficult to communicate with live objects in phase due to their silence or problems with parallel phase retention. However, this is easily solved as you gain experience. In practice, everything looks like this. Let's say you're in a deep phase and decide to find out something about your work partner. To do this, you must use the technique of finding an object and find this very partner. Suppose you leave your room with the thought that he is outside the door. Surely it will, if you do not doubt it. Then, literally, you need to ask him about all the points of interest. You don't need any telepathy or anything. You just need to ask him about it. The object will immediately begin to tell everything, again in a language you understand. No images, visions, assumptions and other subjective. It will be the same conversation as if it happened in everyday life.

During the conversation, you can ask additional and clarifying questions. But you need to remember: if you are a beginner, then you have very little time for the whole conversation (due to difficulties with maintaining the phase), so strive to be concise and demand the same answers until you are brought back to the physical world.

Inanimate Object Technique

In this case, to obtain information from the phase, techniques are used to find objects, which include any inanimate source of information: an inscription, a book, a newspaper, etc. that it will contain or carry the necessary information. You can find a radio or TV and stumble upon the desired thematic programs by switching channels or frequencies. In the phase, you can even use a computer to dig through the search engines, being sure that one of them has the data you need. Of course, my friend, this is the impact of modern technology on the minds of people, but without it, nowhere.

The disadvantage of the technique is that significant difficulties arise when another question appears, or a clarifying question. As a rule, you have to re-find the source of information. However , if the practitioner has trouble communicating with animate objects, this technique may temporarily be a good alternative. At the moment of direct practice, everything can look something like this: having got into a stable deep phase, you focus your attention on the fact that there is a book (or even better - a sheet) in the bookcase, in which the answer to your question is concisely, but essentially stated. Approaching the closet, you must quickly find the desired item on its shelves, which, most likely, really lies there. After that, it remains only to read the contents. If the note cannot be found in the closet or it contains the wrong information, then the whole procedure for finding the object can be done again.

Plot technique

This technique differs significantly from the previous ones . Here you should not find anything. You must move yourself in search of an answer to your question. In some situations, this is much easier to do. Technically, you should just use the teleportation technique with your eyes closed, focusing on the place or object that you need to know something specific about. And you find yourself in a place where you can observe what will be the answer to your question. The advantages of this method lies mainly in the fact that it is better suited for cases when you need to find out the exact events (view them), find a lost object or person, etc. In general, you yourself must decide: when and who is better ask, or read, or see with your own eyes. Let's take an example. Let's say you lost your wallet and can't find it. Having decided to use the phase, you enter it, go deeper and with your eyes closed focus your attention on the thought form of the wallet and the possible place where you lost it (no specifics - just an idea!). Then you will rush in a dark space, and soon you will be thrown to a place where you can observe everything yourself, that is, where you dropped or left your wallet. Naturally, moving techniques need to be mastered here, and this can be an additional barrier to using this technique if there is little experience yet.

Information verification

However, the friend, himself and the techniques for obtaining information are only part of the whole process, as the result may not be reliable. There are only theories to explain why objects sometimes tell the truth, and sometimes lie, honestly looking into their eyes. Some believe that not all information is available. Others believe that certain access may be closed to the practitioner. If we talk about the materialistic position, then the explanation lies in the instability of the properties of objects, which are distorted under the influence of conscious and unconscious thinking, which we will consider separately later. In any case, you need to clearly understand that not everything that you learn in the phase is true. There are several techniques that allow you to deal with this, or at least save you from misinformation.

Clarifying question

The meaning of this information verification technique is simple: in the phase, you need to try to get a simple confirmation of the data from the object by clarifying and additional questions that can prove or disprove the knowledge gained. In other words, you can feel free to demand the whole chain of explanations to be sure of the plausibility. For example, you asked an animate object in the phase if you have any diseases that you know nothing about and that threaten your health. Let's say the subject replied that you have developed a malignant cancerous tumor of the intestine, which gradually grows with metastases. In such a situation, you should not panic, as the alarm may be false. Just ask for some additional facts that would prove such a development of the situation. For example, ask for symptoms.

Linguistic tricks

Any information received in the phase can be partly confirmed by quick verbal formulas. To be precise, they help not so much to confirm the information, but to understand the ability of the object to give out the truth, which is paramount.
There are several such tricks. One of them is that you need to ask a question that has already been answered, just ask it again. This is surprising, but the answer may be exactly the opposite. In this case, naturally, one should be careful not only with the initial answer, but also with the object itself. It is better to find a new object and start all over again. Another trick is to rephrase the same question. Again, in essence, the same question can suddenly have a completely different answer.

Reality Check

Considering that the information received in the phase can have a great effect on the future events of your life, you need to find its confirmation in reality. The more important the information (obtained in the phase), the more actions it implies, the more efforts must be made to confirm it in real life in traditional ways before starting to act. It would seem that this is natural, but many people ignore this approach, forgetting about reason and needlessly trusting the knowledge received from the phase, without having the proper experience to properly handle this resource.

Main difficulty

It can be considered that the ability to receive information from the phase without distortion is a skill, almost of the highest level. What is the problem? As already noted, from a technical point of view, obtaining information does not appear to be anything complicated - it is enough to get into the phase and find out something in it through objects or spaces. Problems arise in a completely different plane, which is much more difficult for a person to control - thinking, attitude, confidence in something, superficial and deep. One of the most interesting and curious tasks, on which work continues all the time, is the study of the dependence of the surrounding space of the phase, its properties and functions on the internal mental background of the practitioner. This task is especially clear in the following example. Let's say that the subconscious mind controls the space of the phase. Let's say a practitioner got into the phase with an indirect technique and rolled out of the body in his room. It turns out that the subconscious mind was able to reproduce this entire room and millions of its small details in perfect accuracy in seconds, in fractions of a second. Is it possible to imagine the amount of calculations that took place in order to create everything at such a speed, down to every thread in the curtains and every dot on the wallpaper, without any errors in physical laws? It's hard to even imagine. Suppose, in this room, a person decided to conduct a well-known test with a calculator, for which he needs to find this computing device and perform calculations on it, which can then be verified in reality. He uses the find technique and finds the calculator. Here again, we note that this is not a certain point in space. This object, even despite its size, is a difficult object, because the phase creates it with unprecedented accuracy and clarity. All lines, buttons, curves - everything is as precise as it is impossible to even draw. Moreover, this calculator can even be disassembled and its device, which was also created together with the entire object in just a few moments, can be viewed. But here's the problem. The practitioner multiplies 34 by 79 and sees some result, for example: AP345V, 59274047 ... etc. That is, anything can happen, but not the correct answer - 2686.

It turns out a paradoxical situation: the subconscious builds space around a person to the point of impossibility, down to its most miserable details, but the same subconscious is not able to multiply two-digit numbers, which is generally possible to solve for the person himself in a few seconds. Does this situation seem strange? In fact, no, Space with its computing resources has nothing to do with it . For him, this is not something that is not a problem - it's just a trifle, even an instant calculation of multiplying hundred-digit numbers by each other. Friend, this is really a trifle for your resource, even if your mind is having difficulty with the multiplication table.

The essence of the problem is in the mind of a person during the execution of this test. He may simply openly doubt the result (and this will be modelled). In addition, there may be a lot of other thoughts and moods in the head that can nullify all the results. For some reason, sometimes it seems that something like this is often related not only to the phase, but also to the ordinary physical world... This situation is very similar to the technique of moving in the phase by teleportation with closed eyes. It is worth thinking about something superfluous, it is worth a little doubt about the outcome of the flight - and it will last much longer, or you will be thrown to a completely different place, or simply returned back to the physical body. When receiving information, exactly the same systems work. But if during teleportation it is enough to move several times to understand the essence, to feel it, then the difficulties with obtaining information are resolved much longer.

There is a proven property of the phase space - it is stable and stable in proportion to the person's perceptions of it. For this reason, the external characteristics of objects can be very stable and unchanging - for example, when in the deep phase you cannot stick your hand into the wall. But at the same time, the properties and invisible functions of these same objects can be very unstable and sensitive to any disturbances of consciousness. That is why it is difficult to instantly evaporate water in the phase or turn it into a blue brick, but at the same time it can be easily turned into vodka, which will be accompanied not only by taste and smell, but even properties, and they will even affect the consciousness of a person if he is will drink. After all, water and vodka look the same on the outside, but differ only in properties. And in the same way, the object created in the phase for receiving information is too dependent on the internal state of the practitioner. The pollution of his consciousness drowns out exactly what he wants to know and what, in fact, objects of the phase can easily give out.

That is why, if you want to receive information in the phase, remember an important thing: not only outwardly, but also inwardly, you must be as indifferent as possible with regard to the information received. In parallel with this, you need to have complete and comprehensive confidence that everything will work out. Without this, the object will oscillate between what you would like to hear and what you are afraid to hear, instead of just giving out information. Indeed, in many ways this problem is solved practically, but there are some tricks that help make the task easier. The simplest of them is as follows: you need to ask the object a question not on the forehead and not immediately, but by chance, during a conversation on abstract topics. This approach simply allows the practitioner to relax and, at least for a while, really remain indifferent to what is happening. Remember this well, my friend, and then work with it in practice if you need it. Although, what does it mean - do you need it? Has someone been prevented by additional information about their loved ones, their work and future?

Case Study

March, 2009
Yesterday afternoon I worked hard on the book, having completed the three-day norm, so the brain was very tired, and he did not have enough night to recover. After working for another hour, from 8 to 9 in the morning, I fell asleep. Waking up before dinner, he ate and again could not resist falling asleep. About an hour or two later , waking up and not moving after a vivid dream accompanied by partial awareness, I realized that my consciousness was quite clear and rested, so I could try to get into the phase, especially since a vivid desire appeared. Tried to split - nothing. I started seeing images. At first it was gray, and somewhere in the distance a forest landscape could be seen again :. He

quickly became more and more real, as if sucking into himself, but I did not wait for this, but once again tried to roll out. The movement was given only a few degrees, and then a dead end. He returned and again rushed to roll out with force. The movement was already much larger , but still a dead end. Once again he returned, with even greater force he began to roll out and did not meet any resistance. I felt that the phase was rather weak. Even deepening techniques hardly helped me. There was no vision, and the degree of stability of sensations was no more than 50% of the everyday world. I was almost pulled back into my body. I had to feel the objects of the room with double diligence, and at the same time practically run around it to add even more sensations. With difficulty, the situation began to improve. When I felt the stability of being in the phase, I raised my hands to my eyes with aggression and tried to examine them through the darkness. They quickly appeared, and the vision covered the entire space and was not inferior in clarity to the vision of the physical world. Since the phase seemed to me anyway unstable and, perhaps, short-lived, I decided not to immediately resort to the action plan, but simply to work on my skills, which I had not used for a long time. First, he went up to the wall and began to bang on it with his knuckles not very hard. Immediately felt an unpleasant sharp pain. He concentrated his attention, and the pain quickly receded. He began to hit even harder. There was no pain. He made a few more blows with all his might, from which the plaster crumbled and a dent appeared in the wall. There was no pain. Then he turned his gaze to the slipper lying near the bed, and tried to move it with his eyes. Reluctantly, with a delay, she nevertheless began to move a little. I noticed that the realism of the space subsided a little, and everything seemed to blur a little, after which the slipper easily obeyed my will. I moved it along the floor, and carried it around the room in the air. As a result, he threw it at the window, which broke; a cold wind blew. Then he lifted the bed up to the ceiling and put it in its place. Then he concentrated his attention on the light bulb, trying to light it with an effort of will. She immediately flared up. By looking and feeling, he increased the depth to hyper-realism and once again tried to light the lamp. It turned out to be more difficult. She didn't really want to obey me. However, after a few seconds, slowly blushing, caught fire. He completed the skill development in the phase by concentrating on the bed cover, wanting to set it on fire. At first, it immediately all smoked. Then , here and there, small flames began to flare up. In a couple of seconds the whole bed was on fire, filling the room with acrid smoke and smell. Rubbing his hands together to maintain the depth of the state, he approached the broken window, not understanding why the phase continues, because it initially seemed unstable. I decided in the last moments to fly in space on some ultra-high-speed apparatus, like those that were in the Star Wars movie. He concentrated his attention on the idea, having previously closed his eyes, and soon felt movement. Gradually, it was replaced by the feeling that I was moving not only myself, but also a comfortable chair (it had just arisen by itself), in which I was drowning. I felt that the body was dressed in some kind of spacesuit, and my gloved hands were holding an aviation joystick. I concentrated my attention on tactile sensations, I was already thinking of creating vision, when suddenly there was a terrible roar and rattle, the Titanic force instantly carried me forward from the chair and what I was in, which was why my body was almost torn to pieces due to seat belts. Unexpectedly, he opened his eyes.

Fortunately, they did not open in the physical plane, and, unfortunately, I saw how, surrounded by sparks, I was approaching a huge spaceship with great speed. There was nothing more he could do. Another second - and around the darkness and weightlessness. Annoyed at the failure of such an interesting adventure, I completely forgot to do anything and soon realized that I was lying in bed, and through my eyelids I saw daylight. I thought it was time to get up and continue writing the book. Without trying to get into the phase again, he went to the bathroom to wash himself, thinking over what had happened . I looked in the mirror and did not immediately understand what was happening: I had a big belly. At first there was a shock, because I spent so much effort to get rid of this "decoration" that arose against the background of strength training. Taking his stomach in his hands, squeezing and rolling thick layers of fat, he realized that this had never even happened before. And then a flash - I'm still in the phase! If anyone knew what a relief it was...

If so, I decided to recall the action plan and, for a start, deal with the structure of the book. I was tormented by doubts about the classification of experiments and their distribution in one or another part of the textbook. The original plan was to discuss this with the subconscious through the sage, but I remembered that the computer with the file open was a few steps from the bathroom, so I went to it, concentrating on the fact that in the table of contents I would see how to line it all up in the best way. He leaned over the computer, opened the folded file. I quickly scrolled through it to the table of contents and saw what was already in reality. This disappointed me a little. I scrolled through the file to the addition, which in reality caused some irritation: everything is somehow awkward and heaped up. To my surprise, I discovered the absence of some sections and immediately realized that everything seemed to be somehow smoothed out, and these sections themselves did not carry anything useful and necessary, although initially they seemed very necessary .

Surprised that the phase was still not over, I decided to try to talk to the sage about the book. With his eyes closed, he focused on him and quickly found himself in the forest near the ancient dolmen. A familiar old man was sitting on one of the stones. Having quickly brought the phase to maximum realism by examining and feeling the hands, blowing on them in parallel, I approached him and asked if I divided the book into parts correctly. The elder, with some kind of cunning squint and an unusual voice for him, replied that it was necessary to describe all the experiments in alphabetical order, and it was not worth dividing the book into parts at all. I did not immediately feel the catch, and for a moment I froze, trying to find a logical explanation for his answer. I suddenly caught myself thinking that I was lying in the body, and immediately all the sensations returned to 100%. He began to try to separate again and apply techniques, but at the same time he analyzed his actions, found them stupid, so there was no chance for separation.

Healing yourself and others

Now, my friend, we will talk about the treatment through the phase and its types. As has been noted many times, the phase state allows you to influence the body, and there are a huge number of options for action. Despite all efforts, this block of knowledge is far from being fully studied. I consider it my merit to single out the easiest and most accessible methods in practice, systematized according to the basic principles of influence. It so happened that I was generally the first who began to study this possibility in great detail and conduct appropriate experiments. And my book on this topic was the first and so far the only work devoted only to this issue. But in this book, I will share with you the most basic principles.

Knowing all the possible techniques and their varieties, you will eventually have to choose a few of the most understandable. However, do not hope that the choice can be made by simple reasoning, only practice is of great importance, that is, how you can do all this. Something may initially sound very tempting, but in the end it will turn out to be difficult, and something will seem the closest, and in real practice, the opposite things will be much more accessible and interesting.

Every time it makes sense to use all possible techniques to influence the body in order to get the maximum effect. That is, one and the same problem should be influenced from all sides, using all possible principles. This approach gives a greater effect, since in case of failure with one technique, the situation will be insured by another, in general, this gives the most correct and stable result. Pay special attention to my comments regarding the availability for beginners of this or that self-healing technique. Of course, the techniques described, as well as specific ones, are not ironclad rules that should never be deviated from. Everything described below should serve as a kind of foundation, a template from which you can build on your personal experience. Perhaps you will adjust or change something for yourself.

Getting Information in a Phase
Action

The meaning of this technique is to obtain useful information that can be used for self-treatment. Moreover, it can concern not only actions in reality, but also actions directly in the phase. You can learn how to help another person, what he needs to do to overcome his illness. For example, having a certain disease or health problem, a practitioner can find out in the phase which medicine is better to be treated in the physical world, or what action in the phase will help get rid of the disease and other misfortunes. The corresponding techniques for obtaining information are described in a separate section of this book.

Indications for use

Indications for use - the most extensive. Since we are talking about gaining knowledge, information, the technique can be applied in any case regarding self-treatment, regardless of the complexity and type of the disease, and regardless of whether you are going to treat it in reality or in a phase.

Example

Let's say you injured your leg at work. A severe bruise causes pain, and healing is slow.

The question arises: what can be done to make the leg heal faster and hurt less? You enter the phase and apply the technique of obtaining information from animate objects, for which you find a surgeon. Briefly describe to him the essence of the problem and ask for advice. Suppose he said that in the phase you first need to run a little, trying to get rid of the pain or simply not feel it, and just before returning to reality, cool your leg with a coolant and inject a large ampoule of novocaine. Also, he can give advice to apply some compresses in reality, which you have never even heard of, or any specific medicines. As a result, all this will remain simple to implement in the phase and in reality, getting the result according to the quality of these actions.

Efficiency

Efficiency (accuracy of the knowledge obtained in this way) very much depends on skill, that is, on the ability to receive information from the phase by the practitioner himself. For a beginner, the number of correct advice may not exceed 20-40%, but with experience, their number can be increased to 70-100%. In this regard, do not forget about the techniques for verifying the information received.

Difficulties

The main difficulty of this type of treatment with the help of the phase is that the practitioner needs to have an additional skill: the ability to get the correct information from the phase and, accordingly, to check it. Usually, you just need to get into the phase and, having gone deeper, perform the planned actions, observing the hold. But in this case, everything is much more complicated. The very accuracy of the acquired knowledge strongly depends on how independent the practitioner is regarding the information received, how confident he is that he can do it. He should not exert internal pressure on the source of information, wanting to hear something specific. That is, the practitioner himself stifles the flow of correct information. These simple things are very difficult to turn off for an ordinary person without serious training, as people are used to thinking about something and wishing for something in the background of consciousness all the time.

Availability

Of course, obtaining information for treatment in the phase or in reality is the most difficult method of all, so it is better for a beginner not to mess with it unless there is an urgent need for it. Unlike many other methods of treatment through the phase, here you need to master a separate and complex skill of obtaining information.

Taking medicines

Action

I think you know the paradoxical effect that taking a chalk pill works exactly as it says on the label a quarter of the time. In the phase, you can perform this trick with much greater efficiency and brilliance, since in it you can reproduce not only any pill (and other dosage forms), but also instantly feel its effect. The body simply has no choice when it has to digest a pill with certain properties. All this makes the body adapt to the events and in reality reproduce the effect in all possible ways. This is a very good method. We are talking about a total deception of the body, forcing it to work in one way or another, solving a specific problem. The key to understanding how this happens lies in the following fact: the body perceives all experiences in the phase state as a reality and on its own in the physical world tries to adjust to the events, reproducing the necessary, missing effect. This is clearly seen in an elementary experiment. If you look from the side at a person who is running in the phase, you can see how his breathing goes astray, his heartbeat quickens, blood pressure rises, and blood may even rush to his legs. And these are only external indicators. At the same time, internal work is going on at the level of secretions, and according to the same scheme, if the run were real. These internal processes can be understood by the following example: drink a glass of vodka in the phase. You will not only smell and taste it, but you will instantly feel the corresponding effect, which can partly be retained even when you return to the waking state. But vodka may not have an effect if, while drinking it, one focuses on the fact that it has the properties of water. That is, vodka itself will lose its properties. That is why, when taking therapeutic agents, one should try to immediately feel them in action, and as strongly as possible.

Self-treatment in the phase through the use of drugs looks like this: the practitioner needs to find (using the techniques of finding objects) certain therapeutic agents or create them, after which they should be taken in the usual way, actively trying to immediately feel the corresponding effect or the one closest to it, if this is impossible. The remedy itself can be of any nature: tablets, pills, tinctures, balms, potions, etc. When a person takes them in a phase, the body begins to reproduce the effect according to his feelings, and in addition, at the level of internal processes, a corresponding reaction takes place, which in the physical world should have been provoked by a therapeutic agent. Everything is simple.

Of essential importance is the ability to create your own medicinal products that have the desired set of properties. For example, you can create and take a pill, when you find it, you programmed the properties to treat two diseases at once or act on an ailment for which there is no cure in the physical world at all. But at the same time, it is worth noting the pattern, which is expressed in the fact that the invented means are less effective due to certain psychological blocks in practicing people. Of course, in most cases, a single dose of therapeutic agents in the phase is not enough , therefore, original treatment courses should be carried out, often in time close to the time as if it were a real medicine. In some difficult situations, as in the physical world, you need to take medicines in the phase regularly throughout your life. If we talk about the doses of therapeutic agents, then one important thing should be noted here: in fact, it was possible not to take drugs at all in the phase, getting the desired effect. It's just that in the phase it is very difficult for a person to force his body to work in the right direction without an auxiliary anchor. The medicines themselves are something with which it is much easier to reproduce the desired self-treatment program. It turns out that the dose does not matter at all, but at the beginning of practice it is better to use impressive norms, since the subconscious program of the influence of quantity on quality will work. But do not overdo it, as a horse dose can cause negative consequences. When the practitioner learns to reproduce the effect of drugs on his own, then it will be possible to use drugs in scanty quantities. There is a good test to understand how to control the properties of drugs, regardless of their quantity. To do this, in the phase, no matter how ridiculous it sounds in the context of self-treatment, you need to take a glass, at the bottom of which there will be 5-10 grams of vodka. If, after drinking it, you can feel the effect of a whole glass (or a whole bottle) of vodka, then you know how to create the desired effect, regardless of the amount. In a similar way, but better with other fluids, buddy, you can just develop this skill in a phase. When choosing various means of treatment, the question may arise: many of them actually have side effects, but will this also manifest itself in the phase? We can confidently say that the effect of side effects is reduced by 50-100%, since for the subconscious, any remedy must first of all treat, and the body may not have a program about side effects at all. Given this situation, it is better not to use drugs whose side effects are well known, since in this case they can not only manifest themselves, but also be dominant in certain technical errors. That is, a drug in the phase can do more harm than cure.

Indications for use

Indications for the use of therapeutic agents in the phase are of maximum importance. As with getting information, it can apply to solving any problem and treating any disease.

Example

Suppose a person has a severe cold, with symptoms; headache, runny nose, cough and fever. He enters a deep phase, finds in it on the table (by the technique of finding objects) an advertised remedy for a quick cure for a cold in the form of a soluble tablet. Immediately he goes to the kitchen and throws it into a glass of water, waiting for it to dissolve. As soon as this happens, he drinks the contents of the glass, trying to immediately feel the effect: warmth spreads through the body, a special feeling of well-being appears, the temperature drops, phlegm and mucus in the nasopharynx disappear, etc. Returning to the physical world, the practitioner immediately feels the effect, or it gradually occurs in the near future. Over the next few days, the procedure is carried out several more times. Then the practitioner can separately conduct a course of treatment in the phase of future colds, so that they occur much less often and less painfully. Of course, as with other points, the technique of finding objects can be applied in a variety of ways. For example, you can immediately find a glass with a dissolved tablet, so as not to waste too much time.

Efficiency

For a beginner, the effectiveness of treatment when taking therapeutic agents in the phase is about 50-75%, that is, in most cases, a bright and stable effect is felt. Considering, for example, that pills are rarely as effective in reality, it turns out that in many cases this is the best treatment available. With experience, efficiency increases to 90-100%. In this case, it is necessary to make an adjustment for the regularity of taking therapeutic agents in the phase, which is often necessary to consolidate the effect.

Difficulties

significant difficulties in taking therapeutic agents in the phase. We need an elementary skill in finding objects and the ability to reproduce their effect during direct reception, which is solved by simply deepening the desire to do this. This is solved, if not on the first try, then on the second or third.

Availability

Medicinal agents in the phase are the main means of influencing the body in this state. Due to the availability and ease of implementation even for beginners, it is this technique that should be adopted in the first place and try to get the result from the very first attempts. This is especially important due to the high efficiency of technology.

Immediate Impact
Action
The direct effect on the organism in the phase is explained by the same effect of its adjustment at all levels under the influence of experiences in the phase, which is described in relation to the technique of taking therapeutic agents. That is, when we do something with our body in a phase, we directly feel the effect there, and, moreover, it really reflects on us in the physical world, as if everything was real. The main difference between the direct impact technique is that the approach to the problem does not go through an intermediary (drug), but directly. In fact, this is a more advanced method, but also more complicated. In practice, everything looks like this. A person enters a phase state and begins to directly influence a diseased organ or organism as a whole with the help of all means that exist and do not exist in the physical world. Moreover, it can affect the body simply at the level of perception, without external contact. It is the feeling of direct impact that is the key factor. Without it, the technique does not make much sense - pay close attention to this.

There are many options for a direct impact on the body as a whole or on its individual parts: heating, cooling, blowing with energy, numbness, massage, injections, ointments, radiation - in general, everything that can and cannot be. In this matter, you need to show initiative and creativity. In the phase, you can influence both the whole organism as a whole and any individual part of it. For example, you can easily warm up your entire body, or you can warm up only the brain or, even more incredible, massage it. It sounds incomprehensible and strange, but in the phase one can really easily put one's hands through oneself, feel for any organ and make the necessary impact. Moreover, this is so realistic that most often a person cannot do this for a long time only out of fear, when he feels that his hand is passing through himself, and with his internal organs he feels how the hand touches them. For example, if a person wants to do something with a liver, then he will not only be able to hold it in his left hand, but at the same time he will directly feel the liver itself and the way he holds it. It is especially scary when exposed to the heart or brain. Phase is the only place where you can do all of this. And these are really just incredible experiences that leave an indelible emotional mark for life. It should be noted that it is possible to influence not only the disease, but also its symptoms. By getting rid of them, you automatically influence their source. This is especially important when this very source is not entirely clear. Of course, as with most other techniques of influencing an organism in a phase, one direct impact is often not enough. As a rule, this needs to be done several times, getting into the phase for several days, or even a whole course of treatment. One way or another, it depends on the skill level of the practitioner in the implementation of this technique; an experienced person needs much fewer procedures than a beginner, but I think this is understandable.

Indications for use

It is easiest to apply a direct effect on the body only in relation to the problem, the localization of which is clear. With direct exposure, it is very difficult to do something with insensible diseases that have few symptoms, the nature of which is not clear.

Example

Consider the first example: a bruised leg. The practitioner enters a deep phase and immediately begins to carry out all possible manipulations on it. Firstly, he focuses on the fact that the leg does not hurt, that it is healthy, and tries to send heat, vibrations through it from the inside, which should produce a healing effect; it must be felt immediately. If there is time left, the person (by finding the object) finds a syringe in which painkillers and medicine are mixed to quickly cure bruises. He injects the entire dose into the leg, trying to immediately feel the effect of the drug, which is easily achieved, that is, the practitioner feels how the numbness and pleasant sensations spread. If possible, in the end, he smears the leg with a special sports ointment, which further accelerates healing. When the practitioner returns from the phase, he will most likely immediately feel that the leg hurts much less, and soon it will begin to recover. But it is desirable to perform this procedure several more times.

Another example: kidney stones. The practitioner enters a deep phase and first, for a minute, tries to "blow out" the kidneys with heat and stone-destroying vibration. To do this, he first tries simply to feel the kidneys, and then, with a strong desire, causes the necessary processes in them. After that, he puts his hands inside himself, gropes for a kidney with each hand and begins to massage them in such a way as if destroying stones in them. Then he carefully puts his fingers into the kidneys and with them grinds the stones into powder. For the greatest effect, the practitioner regularly and persistently carries out the procedure in relation to this particular problem, since it is not quickly resolved.

Efficiency

In most cases, the direct intervention technique is a very effective treatment, especially when the problem is felt and obvious. Even for a beginner, the efficiency can be 60-80%, not to mention more experienced practitioners.

Difficulties

There are no significant difficulties in the direct impact on the body in the phase. You just need to feel a certain effect, which is easy with the proper level of desire, even without prior training. A small problem is the fear of penetrating the hands inside the body, which can be difficult to overcome. But if the goal is serious, then it will be a surmountable task, although for the sake of entertainment you can never dare to do it.

Availability

Direct influence on the disease or problem of the organism in the phase is fairly easy to carry out and, at the same time, very effective. Therefore, even beginners are advised to use this technique from the very first attempts and never forget about it, even after mastering other self-healing techniques in phase states. This is the base.

Programming
Action

As you know, the actions of auto-training, self-programming and self-hypnosis are not questioned even in wakefulness, since these phenomena have long been proven. Their effect is greater, the deeper the trance state in which they are carried out. From this point of view, the idea of using similar techniques in relation to treatment through the phase cannot but come to mind, since the phase state is the deepest hypnotic, trance state that one can achieve independently and consciously. Moreover, the usual trance, in which self-hypnosis is performed, cannot be compared with the phase either in essence or in action. Based on this, self-programming in the phase is also many times more effective than in any other state. In fact, this is a new era in the development of these same technologies. Programming in the phase consists in creating subconscious attitudes that will be carried out independently. Since a person, while in the phase, is in the deepest possible altered state of consciousness, such an impact has the maximum effect. Taking into account the fact that a person invents many diseases for himself and really suffers from this, the programming technique in the phase is able to destroy the root of such "diseases". Directly in practice, a person must get into the phase and introduce into his subconscious mind the attitude to solve this or that health problem. This action in the phase has several options. First, while in the phase, you can simply carefully pronounce aloud the mindset for solving a problem or for feeling well. Secondly, programming can be done without words, at the level of silent understanding and presentation of the goal. This is much more difficult to do and understand than verbal suggestion, so it is better for a beginner not to mess with this option. The duration of one attempt should not take up the entire phase, since the point is not at all in the quantity of efforts, but in their quality. Let it last 10-15 seconds, but it will be brought into the subcortex as deeply and emotionally as possible. Do not think that you can say some words that will work on their own, like a spell. These words must be experienced and felt at all levels of consciousness and perception.

It is very important to note that when programming a verbal formula should not contain negations. For example, you can't say: "I don't have insomnia." Instead, it's much better to say, "My sleep is deep and sound, I fall asleep quickly." And of course, as in other techniques of self-treatment in a phase, in programming it is often not enough to deal with a problem once. It is better to do this several times on different days, and sometimes it is worth taking courses of treatment.

Indications for use

Programming for self-healing in the phase can be applied to almost any disease and illness, but the technique works best for problems related to psychology and general well-being. For example, in this way you can increase your working capacity, endurance, get rid of fatigue and fears, improve overall well-being against the background of an illness, etc.

Example

The practitioner has a serious stage of any disease, which is accompanied by a decline in strength and mood, but at the same time there is no way to lie down, since it is necessary to be present at work. He enters a deep phase and begins to say the following text aloud to himself: "When I leave the phase, I will feel vigorous, healthy, active during the day. I will have a good mood and perfect general well-being. I am well. I am active. I'm happy. I have an abundance of energy and I am full of vitality." At the same time, he not only pronounces these words, but also tries to feel everything, to survive. Of course, before leaving the phase, it is even better for him to carry out additional procedures to treat the disease itself. One way or another, such a suggestion almost immediately upon returning to reality gives a result that can be very stable.

Efficiency

Since most people are not able to fully experience the self-suggested program, the effectiveness of programming for healing through the phase is not very high. For beginners, the figure does not exceed 30-50%. With continued practice, the efficiency increases. Interestingly, in this case, a single exposure is often sufficient , and not multiple, as in other treatments through the phase.

Difficulties

The main difficulty in using programming techniques is the ability to sincerely feel the installation being introduced. For many, due to psychological characteristics and difficulties of understanding, this is an unbearable task. In addition, it should be noted separately the fact that programming can take practice out of the phase itself, since this in itself is relaxation. Therefore, in its implementation, one must not forget to use some kind of holding technique. For example, you can constantly rub your palms together or look at something up close, as well as constantly maintain vibrations.

Availability

Often, treatment in the phase through programming is not easily accessible to beginners, based on the assessment of effectiveness and the difficulties that arise in this case. Therefore, if there is no specific goal that can be solved only in this way, it is better to use other techniques.

Psychological impact

Action
Psychological impact in the phase is the most significant, obvious, understandable and proven way of influencing the body in all cases when it is necessary to solve problems associated with the human psyche and psychosomatic diseases. No wonder this effect in the framework of lucid dreams is recognized by science.

The principles of this technique are extremely simple:
• adaptation or experience of any events in the phase is fully reflected in everyday life;
• a new experience of negative events of the past erases the real physical imprint that they left on the level of physiology.

First of all, it should be noted that the practice of the phase itself, outside the framework of self-treatment, still has a powerful positive effect, which has a very fruitful effect on any person. The point is that, having known the phase (in fact, knowing the new breadth of the world and the absence of horizons), a person begins to relate to real life in a completely different way. He becomes open, less insecure, more sociable. Moreover, the practical conquest of the phase builds some kind of inner core in a person, because this is real work. And of course, how can the practice itself not affect a person, if this is real self-improvement? Real and amazing, and not on the verge of imagination and thinking, as is often the case in many other practices.

Indications for use

What kind of problems are solved with the help of psychological influence in the phase: mental illnesses and disorders (including phobias, fears, complexes, indecision, depression, tightness, and much more). This technique of self-healing in the phase is hardly applicable to any diseases that are not related to human psychology. The exception is ailments caused by psychosomatic causes (according to some sources, up to 50% of all diseases, but it is difficult to single them out on your own).

Example

Let's analyze the situation when a person is afraid to fly on an airplane (aerophobia). To solve this problem, a person needs to get into the deep phase and, using the movement technique, find himself in an airplane flying with strong turbulence. Despite the fact that all this does not happen in the physical world, the fear is 80-120% the same, since the realism of the state is extremely high and there is almost no difference in sensations. But on the other hand, there is no real threat to life, and the practitioner subconsciously understands this, trying to stay on the plane as long as possible, getting used to its rocking, shaking and sharp failures. As a rule, only a couple of such tough simulations of the situation are enough for any phobia, if not to disappear, then recede into the background and stop bothering. Consider another situation - a person who experienced extreme stress in childhood: his beloved puppy died before his eyes. It is in such cases that a chic method works - communication with the spirit of a deceased creature (including a person). This is especially true when, from a technical point of view, there is nothing complicated. You just need to get into the deep phase and apply the technique of finding the object. The puppy will appear exactly the same as it was in childhood. He will also lick his face, play, bark and look at the owner with devoted eyes, wagging his little tail. It will be possible to pick it up again, stroke it, feel its fur, weight and temperature. It will be exactly the same as if a person saw it for real. Even when he bites effortlessly, the owner will immediately feel it. The first such meeting, as a rule, causes some sad emotions and tears, but then, from the understanding that one can continue to see this being in the phase, the problem quickly fades into the background (like all the psychosomatic complications that arose against its background). There is a feeling that this puppy is really alive, because we perceive everything by sensations, and not by conclusions?

Efficiency

The instruments of psychological influence in the phase have a very good effect. Since we are talking about psychology, it is difficult to compare the effectiveness of this technique with other methods of treatment, but even for beginners, success reaches 100% already at the first applications. This is something out of the ordinary in its effect.

Difficulties

Since the object of work with this technique of treatment in the phase is the psyche and consciousness, certain internal efforts are required to achieve the result. For example, if a person tries to overcome claustrophobia, then when immersed in confined spaces in the phase, he will have a real fear, which he will still need to overcome on his own. Here, the phase only provides a springboard for working with oneself. So do not think that the amazing effectiveness of this method is taken from the air.

Availability

Self-treatment in the phase by the technique of psychological influence is easily accessible to beginners from the very first entrances to the phase, since it does not require any special skills, except for the ability to move, so this direction can be used from the very beginning.

Treatment of other people.

My friend, in addition to self-healing, the phase state of the brain provides some opportunities to influence the health of other people. We will consider all possible options, including theoretical ones. It is not news that most people are primarily interested in the issue of not self-treatment, but helping others. It is understandable, because someone has relatives who, for some reason, cannot use the phase themselves or perceive such things extremely negatively, having a stereotyped idea of them. In other cases, the reader of this book may be a non-traditional healing professional or an aspiring healer. First of all, it should be emphasized that out of the whole variety of theoretical ways of influencing another person in the phase, only one is considered proven and obviously applicable. This is getting information. If the effect of all other techniques on the practitioner himself is not questioned and it has been proven experimentally, then the effect of their influence on other people is only a theory that no one has yet been able to prove experimentally. For example, if you find your friend in the phase and give him some medicine, it will have an effect only in theory.

It should be understood that trying to apply everything except the technique of obtaining information is the risk of wasting time and effort. Of course, someone assures that in practice he has proved the possibility of direct influence on another person in the phase. But I will only talk about what everyone can do literally the first time. In all other cases, it can be unequivocally stated: either it is impossible to influence another person, since few people see the result, or it is simply not entirely clear how to do it. One way or another, deciding on such unproven experiments, you act at your own peril and risk. If this can somehow manifest itself, then in practice you yourself will need to understand what exactly needs to be added in order for the impact on another person from the phase to give a stable result. The theoretical attitude to the nature of the phase phenomenon plays a huge role in the choice of actions. If you are a materialist, then, apart from getting information, you will have no other option to help someone. If you allow the occult components of the practice, then there can hardly be any restrictions in the practice itself. This is the choice of each person, but you must understand that even if other techniques allow you to influence other people, the results are clearly not stable, as many question them due to the lack of practical evidence, and not because of their views and theories. That is why I do not say this confidently. The experiments did not give confirmation.

Of course, if you want to help another person, then besides obtaining information, there is another proven way: to convince him to practice the phase, using appropriate self-healing techniques in it. From the point of view of a pragmatic attitude towards the phenomenon, this is a much more correct option than trying to influence a person from the phase. If you decide to cure another person, then the technique of obtaining information will help. It is described in detail in this book, and this is how it can be applied, with the only difference that you must seek knowledge about a particular person, and not about yourself. You can not only find out exactly how to treat a person in reality, but also conduct a comprehensive diagnosis of the body for him. It looks like this: using the technique of obtaining information, you find a specialist who will help you deal with the problem of your person. You talk with this doctor about how to help a person, what can be done in reality, etc. Then you actually reproduce the recipes or advice received from the phase to the person for whom you did all this, or simply pass on the knowledge gained to him. Proceeding from the most materialistic position, one should note the fact that not every person can be helped in the phase. Without going into detailed explanations, I will say: the more you know about a person, the more you can learn about him in the phase. Let's say you've only seen his photograph, then perhaps you'll still learn something about him and somehow be able to help. But if you know this person personally, then the amount of information received about him in the phase will increase dramatically. You need to communicate with a person at least a little before trying to get information about his health and treatment methods that are most suitable for him in the phase.

Theoretical ways to treat others

The methods listed below have not been unambiguously proven in practice. You can experiment with them at your own discretion. If you undertake to help a person in this way, then in no case promise to solve all his problems, because he should not abandon more traditional methods of treatment. Be prudent and realistic about your options, especially if your practice is just beginning and most of the views are based on borrowed theories, and not on your own experience. Also in all techniques you will need the ability to find objects. In order to better understand the essence of the healing techniques of other people, it is important to study them on your own example. This chapter only briefly describes the adaptation of some techniques to others.

Almost everyone will have a question: who are these objects that we find in the phase and treat? This question arises for one simple reason: there are no clear common definitions regarding the nature of the phenomenon itself in order to confidently speak about its particulars. Many (up to 25% of the planet's population) still do not know that the Earth revolves around the Sun, and not vice versa, so what can we say about the phenomenon mentioned ...

Having explained what these objects are, we would find an explanation for the nature of the phenomenon itself. If you are a materialist, then people in the phase, despite their outward realism and authenticity of behavior, are just simulated "clones" that have no connection with real objects. If you are an esoteric, then the object in the phase will be the soul of a real person. Everything is as usual: everyone sees the world in accordance with their knowledge and assumptions. But I always advise you to be careful in such matters, since people very easily fall into the power of delusions of various kinds, from which they cannot then move away for the rest of their lives.

Taking medicines

The adaptation of this technique of treating another person is that it must first be found in the phase (using the techniques of finding). After that, it is necessary, based on the nature of his health problem, to produce appropriate medical treatment, including not only drugs from the pharmacy, but also any possible folk remedies. For example, if he has persistent headaches, he should be given powerful painkillers and other drugs to drink to eliminate the cause (if known) of the symptom.

Immediate Impact

In case of a direct impact on another person, after you find him in the phase, you need to work directly and with emphasis on his problematic organs or on his general state. To do this, you can use both official and folk recipes, various kinds of massages and everything that comes to mind. Suppose a patient has a severe burn. For treatment, among all other options, you can run your hand over damaged skin, restoring it, which is easy to do, or make injections that accelerate healing, use ointments, and so on.

Programming

Having found a person in the phase, you just need to look into his eyes and suggest that he does not have this or that problem, that it passes quickly, that he is healthy, alert, happy, etc. For example, a person has chronic fatigue. In this case, having found him in the phase, you need to convince him that he is full of strength, active, he has an excess of energy, strong motivation, that he is more purposeful, etc. All this must be said in a confident voice "in person" to a person , preferably seeking external changes in its appearance, confirming instant action. You can also get verbal confirmation.

Psychological impact

When adapting this treatment technique in relation to another person, you need to plunge him into the necessary emotions and experiences, after first finding him in the phase. For example, a person is afraid of dogs. Find him using finding techniques, and then put him in a situation where there are many dogs, and they are all friendly to him, caressing and playing. Or, conversely, it can be placed in a situation where the dogs will act very aggressively, trying to bite, but the goal will be for the person to stop worrying and coolly fight off the dogs without feeling fear. Maybe it will not be so easy, but you need to try to change the person's attitude to the situation.

It is also worth noting that this technique can be partly applicable from the point of view of the most pragmatic attitude to the phase. We are talking about the situation when you ask a person to practice the phase. Not to mention those possibilities in self-treatment and other things that it carries in itself, its very presence has an indelible and positive effect on a person. The practice of the phase is one of the most interesting experiences he can ever have.

Case Study
March, 2002
Waking up during the morning multiple awakenings, without moving physically, immediately began to try to

separate from the body. After a couple of seconds, I realized that this would not work now, and began to peer into the emptiness before my eyes, trying to distinguish some images. There was nothing, so after a few seconds he began to do a phantom sway, which manifested itself a little in the legs: both legs went up a little and then went down. This produced a slight tinnitus and a slight "buzz" in the body. Trying to increase the amplitude of movement for 5-10 seconds, I could not achieve anything significant. In order to overcome a kind of barrier, I decided for a while to digress again to the technique of observing images, and then continue the phantom swaying. However, the images arose so strong that I understood: it is better not to switch to phantom swaying, since it is much easier to use a new situation. Some kind of river appeared before my inner gaze, and behind it a steep hill, completely dotted with tall trees. He began to peer, trying to capture the whole picture - from that second it became brighter and clearer. After 2-4 seconds, I realized that I see her as if looking out the window. As soon as I realized this, I immediately rolled out of the body in my room. He quickly got up and began to feel and look at everything. The vision was immediate. The depth was also immediately quite serious, since I saw everything as clearly as in reality. But deepening techniques led to the fact that everything became much clearer and more colorful than I used to see in life. This scared me a little. The thought even flashed through my head to return back to the body, but I was able to overcome myself and immediately concentrated on the tasks set: treating blood pressure, conducting an experiment with the variability of fluids, and a couple of points of elementary mood entertainment. He opened the cabinet door, behind which, in reality, lay a package of medicines. I began to look for some drug in him that would have to cure high blood pressure, or at least help to endure it more easily. Digging in the bag, periodically took out different tubes, packages, jars from it, looking at them to keep them in the phase. At the same time I tried to understand what it is and how much I need it. For a very long time, somewhere within 15-20 seconds, I could not find anything worthwhile. Then he suddenly took out some blue jar of pills. On it was written " LifeMix - life without hypertension. All the best drugs in one. It was very close to what I was looking for, so I immediately took out two tablets, chewed them and then swallowed them. They were damned bitter and nasty. At some point, because of these sensations, I even forgot that I was in the phase and that I must definitely do something so that it would not end. Instead, he leaned over, grimacing and clutching his face in his hands. Suddenly, a strange wave of unusual sensations went through the body. My head and whole face seemed to begin to fill with blood from the inside, causing my lips, nose, cheeks and eyelids to swell. Not to say that it was an unpleasant feeling. It was more unusual. This is especially true of internal sensations in the head. It was as if something was heating up and swelling. At some point I thought I did something wrong. As soon as I thought this, a large bubble filled with cold water burst inside my head. Immediately, the heat was replaced by coolness, and the head and body "shrunk", as if returning to their original state. There was an extraordinary lightness and freshness inside me. There was a feeling that there was a reserve of some kind of strength, resources. In order not to look for this blue jar next time, I put it in the right corner of the bottom shelf. After that, I decided to fix the effect and experience some kind of physical action, which always brought pain in my head from rising pressure. He ran out into the corridor, sat on the floor, pressing his back against one wall, and his feet against the opposite. And he began to push off with his feet, squeezing the wall with his back and thereby simulating physical exertion. At the same time, I tried to look at everything around more, fixing the position, because of which the wall was very tight, and I had to make titanic efforts to somehow straighten my legs. Then I bent them again and tried to straighten them again. I have already experienced physical stresses in the phase more than once, and they were always accompanied by the same sensation of rising pressure in my head, against which sometimes pain arose, and discomfort could even remain in reality when I left the phase. This time there was lightness in my head, and I just concentrated on the physical effort, and not on how hard this process is for me in itself. In addition, I myself tried to consciously remove this heaviness and pressure from my head, trying to set the same program for the physical world. Among other things, he tried to make self-hypnosis whenever possible. Then he began to implement the following points of the action plan ...

Chapter Five

Newbie Experiences

Dear friend, having a database of thousands of descriptions of other people's out-of-body experiences, I want to share some of them with you. Almost all of them will not be the height of perfection, because I want to show you what mistakes people make at the beginning of their journey. This will save you from the same mistakes. Perhaps I approached their analysis too harshly, because it's not always good to ask a beginner like that, especially when he succeeded, albeit not qualitatively. But this is already an achievement. But we're talking about serious things, aren't we? Always rigidly and meticulously analyze your experience and look for all possible errors in it. This is the main secret of perfection. And look for all the mistakes in yourself, and not in anything else.

1. Oksana Ryabova, Moscow, student

My deep morning sleep, as it seemed to me, was interrupted by strong sensations of discomfort and slight pain in my numb left arm, thrown behind my head during sleep. There was a desire to get rid of these feelings. I held out my numb hand in front of me and opened my eyes. But she did not see a physical hand in front of them, although she clearly felt it there and could squeeze and unclench her fingers and bend her arm at the elbow. All this led me to some confusion. Clearly understanding that this could not happen in the ordinary physical world, I decided that this was a very realistic dream and that in order for me to wake up, I just need to close my eyes and strain my brain with the desire to wake up. The thought was followed by action. And after a very short period of time, I opened my eyes and thought that I had finally woken up. Before me was an everyday reality that I constantly observe after waking up: through a large window, sunlight pours onto a bed in the center of the room; desk and chair, shelving: with scientific literature, wardrobe with clothes. Everything as usual. And this midweek weekend, which I have more than days in a week, I decided to spend on a calm, measured rest. I sat up in bed, leaned on bent knees, and, closing my eyes, enjoyed the rays of the May sun falling on me. It was warm and light. And I felt peace flowing through my body like some unearthly sweet nectar. I turned back. And suddenly the state of relaxation was abruptly replaced by cold and trembling, peace turned into a terrible fear - my body lies behind me! Panic. I look at the hands that I feel, but do not see them in front of me, they lie peacefully on the bed along the body. I touch them and feel the velvety of the skin, which I did not feel with physical hands. I'm trying to get back into the body. I lie down in it, close my eyes, straining in an attempt to wake up. I open my eyes, get up, and the body continues to lie. Fear, animal wild fear. Tears. Confusion. Misunderstanding. The question is "What's next?" And all around is that bright day and the sun. And I'm getting more and more scared. The desire to break out of this state increases exponentially. But all my attempts to return to the body are futile. Exhausted and frightened, I sit on the bed like a figurine. And suddenly footsteps are heard in the silence. But I don't see anyone in the room. Fear intensified. And I began to shout to that invisible person wandering around the room so that he would not come near me. Then I ask questions: who is he and what does he need here and why can't I see him?

I get the answer: "Don't be afraid, it's normal." And in a moment he appeared, standing next to my bed. A man with a height of 175-180 cm, about thirty years old, with a dense muscular build. Her hair is short, light brown, her eyes are grey-blue. Was dressed only in black swimming trunks. Around his neck was a thick gold chain. He began to explain something to me about the city of V., calling it a crossing point. Then he said that many people experience such a state and this is a common thing. He took my hand and said "let's go." In a moment we found ourselves in some old city lane. On the corner of the house we were standing in front of, a blue rectangle with the name of the street and the number of the house was clearly visible. I read everything clearly and was surprised by what I saw . We stood in the middle of this lane, almost naked, and people walked past us and did not pay attention. I realized that they did not see us. I kept looking around, shocked and frightened by what was happening. A terrible question for me then kept ringing in my head: how to return? Soon the young man hurried to the corner of the nearest house and, entering the wall, said that it was time for him to return, since his friend was about to come. He disappeared. I continued to stand in the same place for a while, watching people walk past me. I did not know how to get back to my room, because the place from where we came out into the alley was a wall. Here's the problem: how to enter the steppe? Closing my eyes and remembering the room, I stepped forward with my inner motto "whatever happens" and ended up in my bed. Looking around the room, I found that nothing had changed in it, and the sun - it shone just as before. Breathing a sigh of relief and closing my eyes with great hope of awakening, I hurried to open them. And with horror I found a table with medical instruments standing by my bed. A wave of fear swept through the body with renewed vigor. I thought that I would not stand it if they started dissecting me here now. And closing my eyes again, I began to pray. Slowly, the fear subsided, I calmed down ... and finally, I woke up. First of all, I made sure that there was no table with tools, and a moment later, jumping up, I began to knock on the cabinet, on the wall, on the glass - to make sure that it was all really over.

Errors:
1. When awakening, you must first try to separate.
2. Lack of depression immediately after exiting the body.
3. Submission to an unplanned plot.
4. Lack of retention techniques.
5. Lack of a pre-prepared action plan.
6. Deliberate return.
7. Unrecognized false awakening.
8. No attempt to separate again and apply indirect techniques.

Comments: Mistakes are conditional, since the girl did not strive for experience at all - it was the first in her life. It should be noted that an unusually many adventures fell on her head for the first time; invisible hands, unrecognized separation, stranger, travel, false awakening... And all this against a backdrop of horror. The described case once again vividly shows how extraordinarily realistic the experience is - the phase. A person often cannot distinguish it from reality. One cannot ignore the fact that prayer contributed to the cessation of negative experience. The point, of course, is not in the prayer itself, but in the calm that follows. Any relaxation, withdrawal of thoughts inward, allows you to stop the phase. It must also be said that, despite the whole nightmare, this girl later became a very advanced practitioner, since she was very interested in it.

2. Maxim Shvets, Moscow, student

Went to bed with the intention to enter the phase in a dream or in the morning upon awakening, woke up at about 6:30 and decided
to try the visualization method, since the phantom swaying did not lead to anything for two days. Gradually the vague images were filled with a plot, and I myself participated in this plot, felt separation from the body and rolled out. I open my eyes. Some guy grabs me by the shoulders and says: "You are out of the body, be cool." I told him that I was ready. He turned me around by the shoulders, and I saw my body... The body lay on its back with open eyes, although I began to visualize on my stomach. Not attaching any importance to this, I decided to immediately go deeper. He squatted down, began to fluently feel the floor and walls with his palms. Then he looked at his index finger and could see the stripes on it. Deciding that everything was fine, I went to the kitchen, to the window to fly, but remembered that it was better for beginners not to do this. I returned to the door to the room, imagined that there was a sunny beach behind it, opened the door and immediately woke up lying on my back ... This is my first experience. Despite my attempts to go deeper and the belief that I did it, the reality of perception was like in an ordinary dream (I realized this when I woke up in bed), and it seems to me that this was the dream in which I realized the actions, before that many times scrolled in my head. Again, there was no surprise, no shock, etc.

Errors:
1. When awakening, you must first try to separate.
2. You can not try only one technique with indirect techniques.
3. Submission to an unplanned plot.
4. Absence of depression immediately after leaving the body.
5. When deepening, you need to pay more attention to looking after when you already have vision.
6. Insufficient deepening.
7. Lack of a pre-prepared action plan.
8. Lack of concentration when performing the technique of moving through the door.
9. Lack of retention techniques.
10. No attempt to separate again and apply indirect techniques.
Comments: This is a completely typical situation when a person cannot understand how much his experience corresponds to the phase only because the deepening has not been carried out properly. This happens precisely to beginners who have never encountered a full-fledged phase and still cannot understand what it is in principle. Deepening should be done exactly until the degree of realism reaches at least the same level as in everyday life. This probably failed due to insufficient attention to close observation . It can be assumed that when the practitioner saw the lines on the skin of the fingertip, at that moment there was just the same realism that was lacking. It was only necessary to continue this action.

3. Oleg Kudrin, Moscow, manager

Awoke. It was still dark, went down ' till wind ," looked at his watch; 4.15 am. I lay down in bed on my left side, closed my eyes and... It seems that something is shining into my eyes. I am aware that this cannot be: the time is night, and I am the only one who is awake. There is no one else in the apartment, except for the wife sleeping next to him. Meanwhile, the light grew stronger. There was a slight fear, along with curiosity - what will happen next? And then it became brighter and brighter, I felt the danger, but at the same time the instinct of the researcher took over. I will drank that something unusual is happening, because this cannot be - a bright light of an unknown nature hurts the eyes through closed eyelids! Then the thought arose by itself: "They are checking me," and then; "I'll go to the end!"

In the next moment, I found myself in a small rectangular room with subdued light. Along the walls there were ledges (I designated them for myself as benches) on which one could sit. On one of the steps there were round, about a meter in diameter, portholes. Looking into them, I realized that I was in deep space. Outside the room in which I found myself, there was a grandiose construction. What I saw could not have a place in the most transcendent fantasies in ordinary earthly life. It was a truss structure, and its elements did not have a logical structure and from a distance looked like a bird's nest. The design was a double tube of such colossal dimensions that the diameter of only one of these tubes can be compared with the diameter of the stadium. Around this structure, small spaceships scurried and fussed, apparently doing some kind of work. "This is the docking portal," came the answer in my head. I turned around: in the far corner of the room a beautiful girl was sitting, dressed quite according to the earth - in a skirt and jacket. Very strangely, she resembled one famous pop singer, although the resemblance was incomplete. This person was much more interesting. The only question that bothered me at that time, I would put it this way: what is the emptiness that Buddhist teachers talk about? And I asked this question to this pretty lady. For some reason, I didn't think of anything else, and besides, I'm married. However, my question was raised, and it was followed by an answer... What I experienced has no analogues in everyday life, moreover, these feelings cannot be expressed in words - it's just that such concepts do not exist in the language of people, but I will try. It was like the following: it was as if I had been turned inside out, and everything that was outside turned out to be inside me, that is, stars, galaxies, other worlds, in general, the entire material universe. And it all shrunk to such a tiny size that it could fit in the eye of a needle. And I, being outside this material universe, look at it simultaneously from all sides, and I do not have hundreds of millions of eyes, but I am one large field that occupies the space around this shrinking universe, capable of visually embracing it entirely! I myself am infinite, have no boundaries in time and space. There is absolute silence around, and this silence is myself. Contemplating my universe, I came to the realization that with the effort of thought I can turn it into nothing . Next thought: but then there will be nothing to contemplate? After that, it began to collect me, as if into a funnel, from the perimeters of my universe, turning inside it, pulling deeper and deeper, until I ended up on the bed on which I lay down after I went " before the wind". This vision shocked me so much that I could no longer sleep, I just wanted to run outside and jump for joy and delight. I wanted to tell everyone about my experience, just to share, but I thought that they would take me for a schizophrenic. In general, this is how I lived since then, remembering that vivid experience and keeping it in the depths of my soul, dreaming literally every day and hoping to experience this again, until I came across indirect techniques.

Errors:
1. Too active thinking and analysis for direct technique.
2. The absence of independent separation, when there were already signs of a phase.
3 No indentation immediately after leaving the body.
4. Lack of retention techniques.
5. No attempt to separate again and apply indirect techniques.
Comments: Of course, most of the errors can be considered conditional, because the practitioner got what he wanted. But it just worked out so well. He got lucky. He could go on like this and lie in the phase in his body. To achieve regular experience, such actions will definitely not be enough. The experiment also shows an example of obtaining information. It is important to note that the practitioner did not begin to think about where he was and what it was around, but calmly followed his goal. He even sacrificed the opportunity to pay more attention to the girl, which can be very difficult to do in the phase.

4. Artem Arakcheev, Moscow, programmer

He did indirect techniques. When I looked at the images, I saw an episode from a dream that I watched before waking up. The picture was very realistic. It seemed to me that in this dream I could change everything. I tried to get out of the body and instantly flew through my head right into this dream, into the entrance of the house in which I lived as a child. I found myself in front of a window on the second floor. Remembering the deepening technique, I quickly began to examine the window. Then my attention shifted, and I looked at what was outside the window. Everything is in its place, as in life. A man was approaching the door. I don't know why, but I was sure that I should follow him. I automatically flew out of the second floor window, right through the glass. Went down to the level of the first floor. This man came through the door. I followed him, flew through the door and began to pursue him. Then I remembered that I have a plan for (times. At the same moment, the space of the phase began to fade and disappear. I realized that it was worth applying the holding techniques, but I did not have time to do anything. In a moment, I realized myself lying on the bed. Body temperature Respiratory rate and heart rate quickened Repeated attempt at separation did not help.

Errors:
1. Submission to an unplanned plot.
2. Insufficient deepening.
3. Lack of retention techniques.
4. Forgetting a pre-prepared plan of action.
Comments: A typical situation is described, which captures almost all beginners: you don't have or forgot a plan
actions - get involved in the unplanned and
pointless plot. However, one cannot but rejoice that
the practitioner made not so many mistakes, although experience
turned out to be small.   Insufficient deepening confirmed by easy passage through the glass. In the deep phase, objects sometimes acquire even hypertrophied strength, not to mention the usual density for the physical world.

5. Artem Miigazov , Ulyanovsk, student

I am 90% sure that there was a phase (if there was more experience, it would be 100%, but our mind tends to deny everything to one degree or another). It was the day after my first incident. I lay on the couch and tried to use the direct exit. Everything was going well, and suddenly the consciousness turned off for a moment, and when it returned, I realized that I was lying on the bed and I felt a phantom body. I tried to roll out to the side, which, although with difficulty, succeeded. Immediately he began to feel the bed and himself (everything was done in some kind of fuss). There was no sight yet. I decided that I could go deeper and jumped into the floor (more precisely, into the void). It flew not so much and ended up with the neighbors below. Then he flew up to his apartment and stood on the floor. He tried to restore his sight by opening his eyes. It looked like after a big sleep deprivation you try to open them, but they hardly give in. I look: I am standing in my room, and the weather is sunny outside. I decided to try flying (well, I love flying). It turned out to fly up to the ceiling, but immediately began to smoothly fall back and down. Upon contact with the floor, he was pushed up, which was repeated several times (it can be compared to when a balloon falls and hits, flies up and hits again) and only after that was he able to get up. It suddenly became difficult to breathe, and I tried to return to the body, but, of course, I could not. For a moment there was a panic, but then I realized that nothing would come of it and I had to endure it. As soon as I calmed down and relaxed, a foul happened. It felt like it took about a minute.

Errors:
1. Deepening by falling upside down is best used only if the practitioner finds himself in a dark, shapeless space.
2. Insufficient deepening.
3. Creating vision by opening the eyes.
4. Submission to an unplanned plot.
5. Lack of retention techniques.
6. Lack of a pre-prepared action plan.
7. Deliberate return.
8. No attempt to separate again and apply indirect techniques.
Comments: Experience is rather poor. That is why the practitioner had doubts about his identification. On the one hand, the difficult direct technique worked. On the other hand, there are a lot of typical mistakes that are forgivable only when taking into account minimal experience.

6. Dmitry Bolotkov , Moscow, lawyer
When I woke up and began to fall asleep again, the following happened. I was lying on my side and, falling asleep, I saw some vague pictures from the previous dream. And now, my body was filled with heaviness, I practically did not feel it. Here began
light vibrations, I immediately remembered the phase and just relaxed... Imagine my surprise when I felt that I was separating. In the process of separation, the heartbeat became very frequent. So I separated and hung somewhere (I immediately had no vision). Well , I started waving my arms and legs, spinning in the dark, trying to fly away from the body as far as possible. I hit something hard (I think the ceiling). Then I was led to the left, and I took a vertical position. He began to rub his hands, trying to see them. And vision gradually

appeared. I saw my hands, they were smaller than mine in real life, and some kind of greenish tint. Then I saw the situation, it was my old apartment with randomly arranged furniture. I began to touch and examine everything. Everything was very clear, clearer than I see in real life (my vision has deteriorated over the past 2 years). The strange thing was that I felt like my eyes were closed, but I still see. Then I somehow turned off my vision and dived into the floor. For a while I flew down, then I stopped and turned on my vision. I was in space, and I saw completely incomprehensible planets. Since I am afraid of heights, I again turned off my vision and wished to be in another place where there was a solid support. After a while, I felt support under my feet and turned on my vision. I was in the desert, where strange animals were grazing, there were pigeons and scattered chips from the casino everywhere. For some reason I thought I was close to Las Vegas. I walked around there a bit, looked around, and then my vision began to disappear, as if narrowing. And when only a small circle of vision remained, I began to rub my hands and look at them. After a couple of seconds, vision was restored. Then a dove ran up to me, with the clear intention of pecking at my leg, I began to run back and throw sand at it with my foot (I scooped it up with my foot). And then it all ended, I was in the body and opened my eyes.

Errors:
1. When awakening, you must first try to separate.
2. The absence of independent separation, when there were already signs of a phase.
3. Double change of manifesting techniques.
4. The almost complete absence of retention techniques.
5. Lack of a pre-prepared action plan.

6. No attempt to separate again and apply indirect techniques.

Comments: Again, typical beginner mistakes. In fact, the phase was largely random. The practitioner probably lay in it for some time and did nothing sensible, until he was only taken out of the body by chance. What if it wasn't so lucky? A huge number of people suffer because of such untapped opportunities. It is important to pay attention to the widespread incompleteness of techniques. Read carefully: first there were images, then vibrations, then an accidental division into relaxation, similar to falling asleep by force. But it was possible to get into the phase even on images, and even more so on vibrations. No need to change techniques so actively when they show themselves. The experience itself, although not the worst, was most negatively affected by the lack of an action plan, which made it pointless.

7. Roman, Rostov-on-Don, webmaster

My first time getting into a phase. I had a dream in which I was in a hurry somewhere, and at the same time I was constantly thinking. And at one fine moment, I thought that this was a dream, well, I decided to try to get out. I lay down on the ground and began to come out, imagining how I was separated from the body. During the transition, I almost fell out of the phase from stress and fear. But everything went well. The picture is this: the entrance, and I get out of the wall like a quagmire. The feeling of separation was very clear. Suddenly I noticed a man who helped me get out to the end. We met, and he began to tell some details of the world that I got into (I don't remember what he was talking about there, because I looked around and couldn't tear myself away, I was simply fascinated by the world around me). In the end , I became worried about the body and decided that it was time to go back: The return was like a nightmare. Some voices, sounds, incomprehensible sensations. And there was a feeling that time had stopped ... But when I woke up, I was so glad that I could not fall asleep all night.

Errors:
1. Absence of deepening immediately after entering the phase.
2. Illogical behavior - an attempt to get out of the phase into the phase.
3. Submission to an unplanned plot.
4. Lack of retention techniques.
5. Lack of a pre-prepared action plan.
6. Deliberate return.
7. No attempt to separate again and use indirect techniques.
Comments: A very comical case, excusable only because the person did not really know about such a practice yet and this was his first experience. It is comical, because the practitioner, having found himself in the phase through the realization of a dream, was trying to get somewhere else... I cited this case as an example of a very common misconception. If you become aware of yourself in a dream, then your actions should not differ from how you would get into the phase with a direct or indirect technique. Immediately you need to make a deepening, and then implement an action plan, not forgetting about retention.

8. Yan Gvozdev, Moscow, psychologist

During the counting technique, I thought about the park, and the plot of the photograph of the autumn park came to me. I deliberately tried to revive this plot, as if moving its details. I felt inside myself that the state was suitable for attempts to enter the phase, and on the very first attempt I managed to dive into the picture. I ended up in the autumn park, it was very beautiful. For deepening, I began to feel everything around me, leaves, tree bark and my own hands, the condition stabilized, and I went for a walk in this beautiful park, filled with birdsong and freshness of foliage. Since I had no plan in advance, I decided to act according to circumstances. The first thing that came to my mind was the question of how my future house, which I thought about in real life, would look like. I concentrated and by closing my eyes I was transferred to this house. I ended up near a very beautiful building. I didn't even think about such a beautiful house in real life. He went towards him, rubbing his hands along the way to keep his fortune. As I got closer, the debt began to change and take on different forms at the same speed as the thoughts in my head. I was not focused to hold one image, so everything was plastic and changeable, as soon as I turned away somewhere and turned back, the image changed. Then, walking around the house for a while, looking at and touching the furniture, I suddenly thought for a moment that it somehow reminded me of a beautiful hotel, and immediately this house turned into a hotel. Appeared before me as a huge complex of the Egyptian type on the seashore. I entered this huge hotel. It was full of guests. I walked among them, talking to some people and touching them out of curiosity. Then I went towards the restaurant and there I saw a variety of dishes, I tried some dishes. After that, I poisoned myself to continue walking around the hotel, continuing to communicate with oncoming people. Inside myself, I wondered about the near future in real life and tried to understand through whom or through what I could find out at the moment. Suddenly, my wife Alexandria appeared, and together we began to wonder about our near future, it was extremely interesting for us. My wife's doppelgänger behaved exactly like my wife in real life, with the same characteristics. Alexandria offered to have fun and think of something near the sea, for example , to slide down the high slide of the water park, which was located on the territory of the hotel. We climbed the highest hill, already breathtaking. I understood that it is useful to slide down such a huge hill for holding and stabilizing the state of the phase. It was absolutely not clear why the pool below was not visible, where to land. I thought that maybe we should not jump, because it is quite high. But Alexandria jumped first, but I, like a decent gentleman, rushed after her. But here, as I guessed, the hill ended twenty meters from the ground. Asphalt below. There was no time to concentrate and imagine that there was a pool below, and I flew straight into the asphalt. Realism - 110%. While I was still flying, I thought that it must hurt, and with a slap, I landed right on my feet. The pain permeated the whole body, especially the shins and knees. The realization that I had simulated this pain before the fall, just by thinking about it, came immediately, and the pain went away. Then Alexandria decided to have some more fun - she was in a painfully cheerful mood. She found such an attraction cannon that " shoots out " a person straight into the sea and quite far from the coast. My wife again decided to jump first, I immediately followed her. We were thrown far from the shore, we flew 300-400 meters from the shore. While I was flying for Alexandria, I became scared. How is it, in the open sea? Will we swim back to shore? I often have thoughts about the commensuration of the space of the phase and the real, and confusion also happens. Especially with strong realism, you ask yourself the question: where are you at the moment? At such moments, only a deep analysis of the situation with thoughts about the body helps, but this is fraught with fouls. Alexandria was the first to plunge into the water, and I followed her. Due to the fact that the height and speed were high, I went under the water quite deep. There was suffocation. I could not breathe underwater, I began to look for Alexandria with my eyes and saw that she boldly swam down into the abyss of the sea. I became aware and concentrated on breathing underwater. Everything worked out, but the severity of the water and the depths were not left alone. I swam down after her. We sank lower and lower, barely overcoming the water column, to a depth of about 500 meters from the surface. Under the impression of what is seen, all thoughts are sometimes lost, since the events taking place are no different from reality. We swam deeper, and something began to look through. We swam closer and saw something like a cave in a coral reef. A little deeper, the seabed was already clearly visible. We saw a tunnel that led to a cave and headed there. Alexandria seemed to know in advance the whole way. I followed her, not quite understanding where we were going, but absolutely trusting Alexandria. We swam into the cave, passed the water pool and ended up in a rock-type room. The room had windows, like in an aquarium, and you could watch a lot of beautiful fish swimming near this sea cave. There, inside, they met four women who were waiting for a pass and looked like journalists and TV presenters. They seated us across from them. When I sat down on a chair, my movements stopped and I forgot a little. He began to concentrate on questions about our future, forgetting about holding the phase. When the dialogue started, I started asking them my questions, and at that moment I accidentally thought about the body, and the foul followed. But still, I received a lot of visual information, which I later sorted out according to images and events. Soon, two weeks later, in real life, I went to rest in a large hotel, where I observed the same images that were described above in this phase. Of course, the coincidences were not 100%, but the overall picture of the situation absolutely coincided in meaning and significance.

Errors:
1. Submission to an unplanned plot.
2. Lack of a pre-prepared action plan.
3. Overthinking.
4. No attempt to separate again and apply indirect techniques.
Comments: This experience, of course, cannot be called amateurish. The understanding of all the most important aspects of the practice of the phase constantly shows through: deepening, retention, application. But why did the practitioner simply obey the events, understanding their essence? This question arises only for those who have never been in the phase. From the outside it seems that the application for real life purposes is the main thing. But in reality the experience is so interesting in itself, so colorful and realistic, that often you don't want anything from it. You just enjoy it. And you don't need anything else.

9. Dmitry Plotnik, Moscow, engineer

Upon returning from an evening walk, our legs took us to the Magic Stone store. There we purchased a stone thing called a druse (an accumulation of crystals on a stone substrate, in our case, amethysts). According to I., this thing must somehow "tune dreams." To do this, the druse should be put at the head and just go to bed. So we did. In the morning we had to get up at about 5 o'clock to catch the tour. We didn't have time for what is called "kolobrodit", but I still tried to tune in to the dream. At some point, I fell asleep, but continued to have a dream that I was lying on the couch and trying to tune in to the exit. At that moment, I felt a slight impact in the back area, as if from some kind of creature. I further mentally supported him, thinking: "Well, come on, so act!" The sensations began to intensify, now they resembled waves sliding along the back. At the same time, a characteristic sensation was going on all over my body, already quite forgotten by me. The sensation could not be called pleasant in any way, and I also thought: "Now it is clear why I stopped consciously striving for the phase." However, it was too late to retreat, and at some point I was carried upwards, I only had time to look back at the sofa. The next moment I was in a spacious room. It was so large that I could clearly see only the wall closest to me. There were also some people in the room. They all wanted something from me and constantly climbed up to me with various stupid claims, but I regularly "shushed" them, trying to drive them away. There was only one thought in my head: "I must find I.". I directed all my efforts to remembering the place where we fell asleep together, but my memory did not want to help me. At the same time, I was constantly distracted by various characters, one of them was especially persistent. At one point, he even pestered me with a request to open a bottle of wine for him with a corkscrew. I decided to help, and when I opened the bottle, I thought: "What the hell?! I have never tasted wine in a phase!" - and applied directly to the neck. The wine turned out to be rather strange in taste, more like chokeberry jam diluted in water , with small particles of berries. The unfinished bottle from my hand disappeared somewhere, and I continued trying to get out of this room. In the recess of the only wall I could reach, there was a strange structure made of wooden boards, painted as if with oil paint (most of all it looked like a huge toilet). I was poking around there, but the persistent character: warned me that "..this is a portal from where uninvited guests can flood ...". I myself did not burn with the desire to climb there and limited myself to removing a small muddy mirror from the outer wall of the building. I fooled around a bit with my reflection (which didn't always follow my movements), but the clingy characters didn't want to be left behind. Then I decided to entertain them a little, and we began to look into this mirror for a couple, in turn with each. And in the mirror they were very different from the "real". I quickly got tired of it, and I again dispersed everyone. In the end, I decided to leave this building, concentrating on the possible setting of our sleeping quarters. I abruptly opened the door, but was disappointed, outside was an unfamiliar street setting. It looked like it was early morning in the yard, rather gloomy, lonely cars were rushing through the street. I began to look at the cars parked on the side of the road. They looked pretty interesting. Suddenly, another car swerved off the street towards me. She drove up to me, and I saw an interesting woman sitting behind the wheel. Her clothes were mostly green. We started talking, and I constantly had the idea that she was speaking as if by writing , as if she was quoting a book. I told her so: "Now you will say such and such ..." She looked at me, and I noticed her strange eyes. Instead of normal pupils, she had green ladybugs. I realized that I was beginning to return to reality. Woke up. I realized that I was lying on my back, my arms along my body, in my left palm I carefully hold the palm of I. I try to remember how I managed to fall asleep like that, but I can't. I remember falling asleep in a different position. I began to restore memories of a lucid dream and I understand that something does not fit. My memory persistently tells me that in addition to a lucid dream, I also had a simple dream at the same time about the same house from which I left at the end. In this dream, I looked at the house from the side for a long time, I was surprised at its large size, its high outer columns. In a dream, this house belonged to N., but I did not understand how such a "rich woman like N." (since he lives in such an expensive house), can meet such a "poor guy like me." In this dream, I went into the house, saw N., saw that N.'s guests were drinking champagne and having fun. I felt uncomfortable in this expensive environment. I lay in the dark and tried to link together these two contradictory facts. Suddenly, N. woke up and began to tell her experience ...

Errors:
1. When awakening, you must first try to separate.
2. Lack of controlled separation.
3. Lack of depression immediately after leaving the body. 4 Submission to an unplanned plot.
4. Lack of retention techniques.
5. Insufficient concentration when performing the technique of moving through the door.
6. No attempt to separate again and apply indirect techniques.
Comments: Although this experience is quite interesting, loaded with a number of curious events, its main feature lies in a completely different plane. Believe it or not, that same "stone contraption", Druse, really

worked. Firstly, the practitioner himself is familiar to me, and before that, he hadn't succeeded in anything sensible for a very long time. Secondly, he is familiar to me through the same N., whom he was looking for in the phase and could not find. This N. is one of my most successful students. But the point is not even that, but the fact that she had her own experience almost at the same time. This is the rarest case when two close people, being together, almost at the same moment independently enter the phase. The next experience just belongs to the second half.

10. Nadezhda Maslova, Moscow, designer

The night it happened was very restless, as we had to wake up early to go on a tour and were afraid to oversleep. I woke up several times in the middle of the night and finally decided to use my awakenings and get into the phase. I successfully made the "exit" and got up from the couch. I was in the same room in which I fell asleep, but found that two mirrors were hanging on the walls, which were not in reality. I looked into one of them and saw that I was wearing the wrong clothes in which I fell asleep. Then I remembered my fix idea - to pull my young man into my phase. I go to the sofa, drag him by the arm, and then start pushing him to the mirror. Then I thought: "What if he sees himself in the mirror and becomes aware in my phase?"
We stand in front of the mirror, and I see that our images are blurred in it. Then I decided that nothing worked out for me again, and let him go. And she herself decided to climb into the mirror in order to move. I climb onto the table, put my hand into the mirror first, and then my head, and I understand that the mirror is "closed" - there is blackness and a wall behind it,

because of this it is impossible to move anywhere. Then I decided to use the "rotation" technique. I unwinded and began to imagine the birch forest I liked from one of my journeys in the phase. I really wanted to go there again. I was spinning and spinning, but I never got into the forest, although it clearly flashed a mile of my eyes, only I could not stop in time. But I ended up in my mom's apartment. I look - a toy hare lies on the floor. I took it in my hands, I think that if I start to lose the phase, I will fiddle with it in my hands in order to gain a foothold. Then I again saw a mirror on the wall and decided to look at myself. I look, and it's not me, but some vague creature that looks like a ghost. I then got a little scared. Because of this fright, I was returned back to my body (I thought so in the phase), and with a hare in my hands.

I ended up in my bed again, but I didn't calm down. I decided to try another way to get my friend into the phase (well, it's boring for me to wander there alone!). I wrapped my arms around him and rolled out of bed. And we really fell off the couch, but not on the floor, but as if we had fallen from a hill, and so we hung in the air. The room we slept in was dark, and we fell during the day, and everything around was very bright, obviously brighter than in the previous story. Well , finally, I think I managed to pull him into the phase! And then I see that the hands that hug me are clearly not his. I look up and see that I am cuddling with another man! In some ways, he looks like my friend, his face is older and a little different, and his hair is long and in a ponytail. I push him away from me and ask: "Who are you?" And he answers me: "Well, I already told you my name. Or maybe you just see the future? I calmed down a little and told him: "I need a dress, I don't want to run half-naked." He says: "Come on, let's buy." I turn around and see the store. We go there, or rather, we fly about thirty centimeters above the ground. We are met by a young mulatto salesman who shows me dresses hanging on hangers. I am delighted! I'm heading towards them... and then I find myself back in the body! It was such a shame to wear such chic dresses at least in the phase!

Errors:
1. Absence of depression immediately after leaving the body.
2. Lack of concentration when performing the technique of moving through the door.
3. Submission to an unplanned plot.
4. No attempt to separate again and apply indirect techniques.
Comments: It will be interesting to know that Nadezhda and Dimitri subsequently married. Of course, I personally do not think that the matter is in the druze itself. I think it's about people's belief that it should work. It became a kind of program. For some reason, it is very difficult for a person to express intention clearly. Very often you need something else physical, personifying your desire and will. And the main mastery of this life is to learn to express your intention as effectively as in the case of this druze, but without external objects and actions. Whoever learns this, not only the phase will open, but also all the other treasures of earthly life... Well, my friend, during our communication in this book, we got to know each other quite well. You know almost everything about my inner world. But don't think that since I haven't heard a word from you, I don't know you at all. No, I know what you were thinking when you read my lines. I know what emotions it caused in you. And I know that now in the heart of both of us there is something in common that

cannot but make us related. We are now close friends. And since it happened so, then I have no choice but to wish my inquisitive friend good luck in his journey. I tried to show you everything at the highest level, although I omitted most of the details and my knowledge so that you would not completely get confused. I hope our acquaintance will be useful to both of us, that it was not in vain. For it to be so, you just need to open a new life with the help of a phase. Good luck!